Dedicated to my wife Valerie

for her support and tolerance

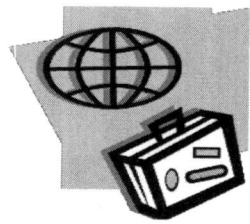

Travel and health in older people

A Guide for Health Professionals

I B McIntosh.BA(Hons).MBChB.DGMRC.DRCOG.FFTMRCPS(Glas)

Publisher

IMCI Publications and Research

2011

Copyright

Front Cover : Pamela McIntosh

Illustrations : Valerie McIntosh

Preface from the President of British Travel Health Association

Providing care and advice for the elderly traveller often seems to be a neglected aspect of travel medicine. There is very little literature specifically on this topic. It is surprising that more is not written since international travel by the elderly is now very common and increasing. Every General Practitioner, Practice Nurse and Pharmacist involved in giving travel health advice will know this all too well and will see elderly patients regularly. This may be because the issues involved overlap a variety of professional specialties. All the usual concerns apply such as determining appropriate vaccinations schedules and malaria prevention.

However many, probably most, elderly patients have a background history of present or past medical problems, which need be taken into account when they are planning their trips quite apart from the issues arising, for example, out of the normal physiological and mobility changes associated with aging. Sometimes experience helps the elderly traveller to avoid risky situations but this is not always the case. A large number of the elderly are on multiple medications and availability may be an important issue to address. Side-effects may occur while they are away in unfamiliar environmental surroundings or undertaking unusual activities. Some are on drugs which need blood test monitoring such as anticoagulants. Medical care abroad may be difficult to obtain and health insurance sometimes be difficult to obtain or very expensive. All these factors explain the need for more training and professional support for those advising the elderly traveller and this book has been a leading resource on the subject for many years.

It has recently been updated and can be strongly recommended as an important and reliable reference on the subject as well as being an enjoyable read.

Eric Walker MBChB,DSc (Hon Madras),FRCP. FFTM (Glas),

Authors

Julie Gallagher

MBChB. DTM. MFTMRCPS(Glas)

General Practitioner. Has travelled extensively and runs an Adventure and Tourism Travel Health Clinic in Edinburgh. Former work in several Infectious Diseases units in Scotland, in the field in Africa and Asia and doctor for commercial companies and Youth Development charity, Fulcrum Challenge. Founding Director of the Alliance for Rabies Control. Chair of executive committee of the British Travel Health Association, and Editor of the Association's publication Travel Wise.

Iain B. McIntosh

BA(Hons). MBCHB.DRCOG. DGMRCP. FFTMRCPS(Glas).FBSMDH

Author of several books, chapters and many research and general papers on travel related medicine. Co-founder, past Chairman, current President and Fellow of the British Travel Health Association. Editor in Chief of the association journal and Travel Wise. Former editor of Scottish Medicine and Rostrum. Editorial Board member Geriatric Medicine. Former General Practitioner, trainer and Hospital Practitioner(geriatrics).Established one of first Scottish travel health-related clinics and national conferences. International lecturer to public and professionals on travel health topics. Extensive travel experience over seven continents. Expedition doctor, air repatriation physician and travel health consultant.

Larry Goodyer

BPharm, MPharm, PhD ,MRPharmS, MFTMRCPS (Glas.)

Professor of Pharmacy Practice and Head of School of Pharmacy, De Montfort University, UK. Clinical pharmacist and until 2003, was head of the pharmacy practice group,King's College London. Principal interest in travel medicine and promotion of role of pharmacists. Lectures on Travel Medicine to Health professionals and public, addressing National and International Conferences television and radio audiences. Deputy Chair,British Travel Health Association, committee member Pharmacist Professional Group of International Society of Travel Medicine. Involved in research on wide range of issues related to the Profession of Pharmacy, including new roles for pharmacists such as prescribing and medicines management.

George Kassianos –

MD (Hons), FRCGP, FESC, DRCOG, LRCP (Edin.), LRCS (Edin.), LRCP&S (Glas), DMedAcup., DMedHypn., DFP, FFTM RCPS (Glas)

An Executive Partner in general practice. Current Editor-in-Chief of the international journal Drugs in Context and past editor of the Audit in General Practice journal, Care of the Elderly, and Managing Heart Failure in General Practice. Founder Member, Spokesperson, Fellow & Hon. Secretary of 'The British Travel Health Association' , Member of the Department of Health National Child Health Immunisation Programme Board, and the JCVI's Hepatitis B Group spokesperson on Immunisation for the Royal College of General Practitioners member of the National Travel Health & Network Centre Advisory Board and The Health Protection Agency's Advisory Committee on Malaria Prevention in UK Travellers.

Mike Townend

MB, ChB (Hons), Dip.Trav Med. FFTM RCPS (Glas))

Former GP, with a travel health clinic. Travel includes Himalayan expeditions and overland to India and leading tours in India, Nepal, Bhutan, Southeast Asia and South America, ranging from mountain trekking to white water rafting. Travel related publications include, traveller's diarrhoea, acute mountain sickness, trekkers' health and asthma at high altitude. Lecturer, Glasgow Diploma, Diploma in Mountain Medicine Expedition Medicine courses and ran a Travel Medicine course in Lancaster. Has written two books on Travel Medicine and contributed to others and articles, for medical and nursing publications.
Founder member of BTHA,member of its Executive Committee.Co-editor of Travelwise and chair of Publications subcommittee, Member of the International Society of Travel Medicine and International Society for Mountain Medicine.

Acknowledgements

Thanks for support with this project from:-

British Travel Health Association

Monument Press. Stirling

and appreciation for IT support from

Gordon Robertson,June Macdonald and Colette Martin

Contents

Travel and Health in Older People

A Guide for Health Professionals

Chapter One

The Effects of Ageing on the Traveller

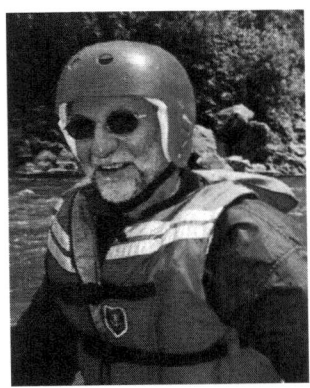

Older people make up an increasing proportion of the UK European and North American populations. Many lead active and healthy lives for many years over the age of 65 years. With increasing life expectancy there will be many more of them, motivated to expand personal horizons and fit to embark on travel. Living longer, they can anticipate years of international travel after retirement from work. In Britain the number of elderly people and pensioners is increasing steadily each year. Soon twenty per cent of the United Kingdom population will be 65 years of age, with a considerable increase in those over 75 years. anticipated in coming years. By the year 2010, 7.2% of the population will be over that age. 1

Life expectancy Table 1

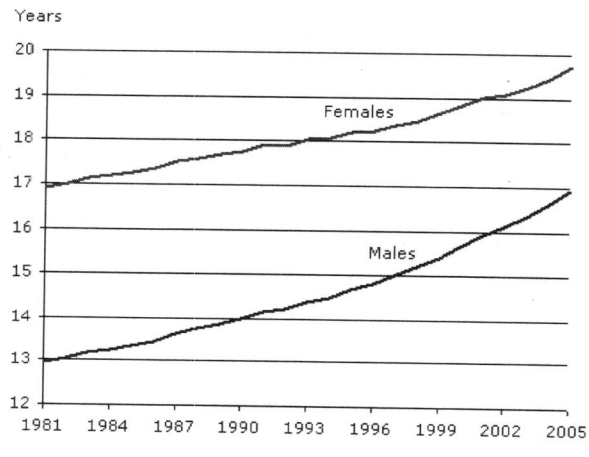

Years

Life expectancy at age 65, United Kingdom

Source: Office for National Statistics; Government Actuary's Department

Life expectancy at age 65 in the UK has reached its highest level ever for both men and women. Men aged 65 can expect to live a further 16.9 years and women a further 19.7 years if mortality rates remain the same as they were in 2004-06.[2]

The majority of the recently retired population are physically fit and in good health. They have time on hand, relative affluence and past experience of travel in near Europe. A large number are now seizing the opportunity for extensive travel abroad. Budget and no-frills air travel encourages them to make long-anticipated global journeys of a lifetime, to meet loved ones and satisfy a thirst to see the worlds wonders and enjoy international adventure before passing years bring declining health. There is a window of opportunity for people aged between 65 and 85 years to travel to the far corners of the earth and many now do so regularly. The majority of older people make the pilgrimage to distant family and fulfil world travel dreams to remote objectives without mishap. With women having a longer life expectancy than men they will travel into more senior years and widowed, many may choose to travel on their own.

United Kingdom Population

Table 2

Over 65years of age.		Life expectancy, years.
	Women	men
2008	20.1	17.4
2009	20.3	17.6
2010	20.4	17.8
2011	20.6	18.0
2012	20.8	18.2
2013	20.9	18.3
2014	21.1	18.5
2015	21.2	18.6

Source: Office for National Statistics; Government Actuary's Department

Not only can they expect to live longer, many can also assume that they will remain physically fit for much of this time. The majority will remain healthy enough to undertake global travel to the farthest reaches of the planet in the first decade after current state retirement age.

Health Expectancy: Living longer, with years in good health
Table 3 Source: Office for National Statistics; Government Actuary's Department

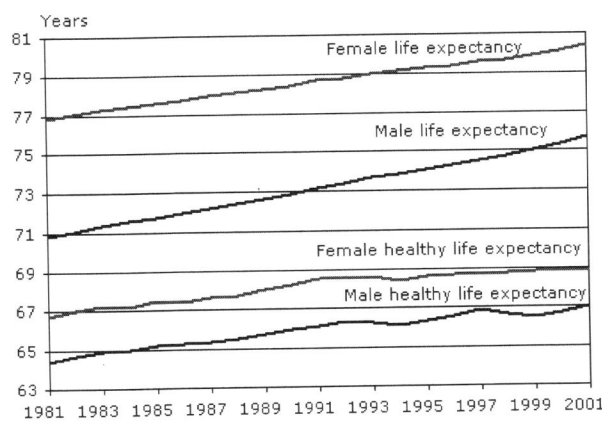

The healthy and not so well depart from Britain on vacation and intercontinental journeys, often with scant concern or consideration for risk to health that world travel can bring. They travel to destinations in undeveloped countries and to remote parts where conventional medical support in emergency is not available. They venture forth undeterred by pre-existing and chronic illness and on medication and can put their lives at risk .Few consider the availability and quality of local medical resources and repatriation possibilities when embarking on eagerly awaited holidays.

Many depend on travel medical insurance cover for protection in time of need. This cover may be illusory however and is limited to the best available in the locale, is dependent upon the environmental factors and may not match needs in an emergency. Insurers are becoming more selective in accepting senior citizens as clients and some older people are now travelling with limited or no health insurance protection. If medical emergency arises while they are away and immediate first aid is delayed, local resources can be inadequate, evacuation protracted and hospitalisation sub-optimal. This may have a serious impact on the individual and their recovery. Chronic morbidity and mortality is a possibility and in the absence of adequate health insurance protection financial demands for treatment and repatriation may prove penal.

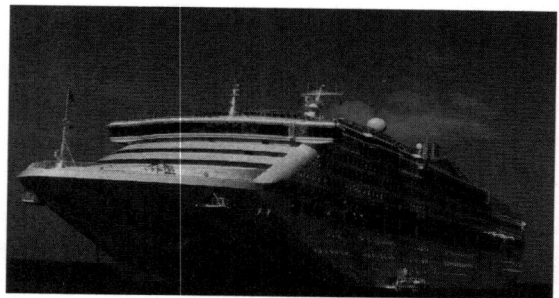

Case History
An unfortunate cruise ship experience
A 72 year old man who had previously had a myocardial infarction and transient ischaemic attacks was determined to continue his winter cruise ship voyages in the Caribbean Sea He was unable to obtain travel health insurance cover for his cardiac condition and stroke disease and opted to travel uninsured. He made one trip without medical mishap and on the next voyage suffered a severe stroke on board ship. He was disembarked at the next port of call on the island of St. Thomas and ultimately transferred to hospital in the United States. His medical and nursing care fees were exorbitant and meeting them bankrupted the family. The endeavour to meet fees and care for her husband precipitated depressive and physical illness in the spouse, who required hospitalisation herself when the patient finally returned to the UK. Many elderly travellers conditioned to NHS care do not appreciate the high cost of health support overseas.

Physical and clinical fitness.A large number of elderly people remain fit and well into their eighties and can indulge in international visits and holidays with impunity. Many retain car driving ability into advanced old age-a measure of their independence and capability.

UK.Car driving licence holders: Table 4

Gender	years	years	Percentages
	50-9	60-9	70 and over
Men			
1996/1998	88	82	64
1999/2001	88	86	69
2002	89	85	68
Women			
1996/1998	63	48	20
1999/2001	69	57	25
2002	74	56	28

Source: National Travel Survey. Dept. for Transport UK.

Community surveys have shown that 80% of 75 year olds are fit enough to travel from home unassisted and considerable numbers now indulge in international travel.[3] In a community study of people over 65 years old, 33 percent had travelled out with the UK within the past year and 35 percent of 75-80 year olds had participated in foreign travel, in the preceding 3 year period.[4] Many elderly people set off from the security of their homes and the protective net of the NHS and reciprocal European Union health provisions on long foreign journeys, ignorant of the health risks which accompany global travel. Seeking winter sun and relaxation they embark on world sea cruises and the increasing popularity of fly/cruising and adventure holidays is testimony to their commitment to far distant travel.

In Britain, many now take early retirement at 60 years age, or leave employment aged 65, assuming maintained good health until well into their seventh decade. Statistically many can anticipate healthy global wanderings until the mid-seventies with serenity.[5]

Thereafter, increasing age and chronic disease begins to take an inevitable toll and may make long distance travel a more hazardous undertaking. The stereotyped view of the elderly person as confused, disabled and dependent is outdated and one finds elderly people exploring in the Amazon, visiting polar regions, climbing to high altitude and adventuring into remote parts of the world. They are also more likely to indulge in active leisure time activity while abroad and participate in white water rafting, para-gliding, snorkelling and horse riding intent on making up for lack of opportunity when young.

Mild and moderate physical impairment does not deprive the right of the elderly to venture afar or indulge in active sports, but they should do so with careful consideration of potential additional risk to well-being. It is the responsibility of the health professional and the travel agent to apprise them of likely health hazards they may encounter when far distant from home. They should endeavour to minimise the risk and optimise protection. General Practitioner, surgery nurse, and practice travel clinic pre travel encounters with intending travellers are ideal opportunities to meet this challenge.

Ageism and age discrimination are still dominant attitudes in Britain. Many cultures value their old but Britain has yet to come to terms with its elderly population and value their contribution to society. There is often an assumption that advancing years alone rob the individual of physical and mental prowess and steal away independence. Compensatory mechanisms, the accrued wisdom of years and sound medical advice can, however ensure that most of older global holidaymakers will travel in good health.

Realistic recognition of the wear and tear effects that come with advancing age is a prerequisite for enlightened risk assessment of foreign travel in senior citizens. The fittest and most healthy older traveller has not the physical integrity or endurance of those in the prime of life.

Reduction in immune, renal, cardiac and pulmonary function and declining glucose tolerance with physiological stress can place the elderly at higher risk of succumbing to travel-induced illness Pre-existing disease, plus the effects of senescence, can make senior citizens` very vulnerable to ill health during international travel. Mild mental and memory impairment can precipitate confusion in stressful travel situations. As a cohort they are also more likely to have an impediment of physical disability which has to be considered in travel abroad.

Health status and the traveller.

In terms of health risk, the potential older traveller is likely to fall into one of three categories:[1]

1. **The low risk group** - the 'young' old includes those :-
   - travelling to low risk destinations;

   - on short-haul journeys;

   - free from any pre-disposing illness

2. **The medium risk group** includes:-
   group 1, where travel involves environmental extremes, or tropical countries;

   - the frail old-

   - those with pre-existing illness

3. **The high risk group:** -

   - the terminally ill;

- those :-on "last-fling" holidays with terminal illness.

    with pre-existing illness travelling to high-risk countries.

    with pre-existing illness visiting areas:-

        with environmental extremes

        in the tropics.[4]

Aeroplanes, cruise ships and tourist resorts will have their complement of older people in all of these categories who will enjoy their vacation and return home in sound health. A minority will however become ill abroad, require local medical services, evacuation and repatriation. Some will never return to good health after acquiring travel induced illness and the experience will prove physically and psychologically traumatic. This critical event may adversely also affect the travelling companion and spouse.

Effects of the ageing process.

The 65 + years age group of people shows differences from the general population and younger cohorts, which can have an effect on the outcome of global travel. [6]

These are:-

- Heterogeneity of health status

- Age-related physiological changes

- Increased incidence of co-morbidity

- Atypical disease presentations

- Increased incidence of iatrogenic illness

- Higher need of social support

- Functional disability increases with age and is closely associated with chronic disease [6]

Pre-existing or chronic illness is likely to affect this group and had to be considered by travel health professionals when they travel far from Britain. Long term illness and disability affects an increasing number of people with advancing longevity.

Long-term illness or disability which restricts daily activities: by sex and age

Great Britain		Percentages
Years of age	Men	Women
50-64	27.02	26.44
65-84	47.22	47.57
85 and over	67.10	73.79

Limiting long-term illness: calculated from a 'Yes' response to the question Do you have any long-term illness, health problem or disability which limits your activities or the work you can do?' This includes problems due to old age

Source: Census, April 2001, Office for National Statistics General Register Office, Scotland

Many people in the older age group are however healthy, health-conscious and follow active fitness programmes. They still wish to travel and they should be encouraged to do so as long as it is practical, but the impact of relocation, international transit and environmental factors en route and at the destination require consideration. The medical risk factors of transit mode, destination, itinerary, local environment and the medical facilities at the locale require the attention of a knowledgeable doctor or nurse. This requires pre-travel health consultation when clinical assessment, risk, precautions and prophylaxis can be discussed.

Age in years is not the arbiter of fitness to travel abroad, however a fit ninety year old will have a pulmonary function only half that of a thirty year old,[7a] serious consideration when the individual can be exposed to reduced partial pressure of oxygen in an aircraft, or at high terrestrial altitude.

Effects of the ageing process impacting on the world traveller [8]

Changes occur in:

Renal function

Water and sodium regulation

Temperature regulation

Cardio-pulmonary function

Gastro-intestinal function

Cell-mediated immune response

14

Changes also occur in

Neurological function

Metabolic response [8]

The physiological baseline in the older individual should be considered by health professional and travel organisers, so that advice can be given on health risks likely to impact on their travels.

Physiological function effects.

Renal function

60% loss of renal function by age of 65years

decreased :-sodium conservation

ability to conserve water

sweating ability

pulmonary function

ventilatory response to hypoxia

increased cardiac load [6,7,8]

Psychological factors also require consideration in the long distance international traveller. The effects of stress in airports and transit stations and congestion on the roads and public concourses can be marked in the general public and have deleterious health effects in elderly people. Transit through airport lounges has been shown to have marked physiological and psychological effects on travellers [9] and may be sufficient to tip the vulnerable older person into cardiac failure or arrest.[6]

When the potential adverse effects of over-exposure to the sun, tropical infection, high altitude and environmental effects are also considered, it is obvious that there can be disadvantageous effects on global travellers' health status. Many of these can be neutralised by careful advance planning by traveller, travel health professional and travel agent organiser.

Following Chapters. The following chapters in this book, contributed by experts in travel related medicine consider:-

risk assessment ,

travel-related health hazards ,

prophylaxis and precautions ,

effects of differing transportation modes,

adverse environmental extremes,

pre-existing illness in world travellers.

Assessment procedures, vaccination schedules and therapeutic procedures are presented with emphasis on the practical handling of potential older travellers in travel health consultation and the travel health clinic. Chapters on sea, air and adventure travel identify risk and offer recommendations to minimise hazard. The diabetic, cardio and pulmonary and immuno-compromised traveller is dealt with in depth.

This medical hand-book is a comprehensive aid which should assist all involved in travel-related health care of older travellers. Its advice and recommendations can ensure that older people, who seek a pre- travel health consultation, will travel aware of risk and take appropriate measures to reduce it and this should ensure they travel and return in sound health.

References.

1 Office for National Statistics . 2007 Govt. Actuaries Dept.
2 Travel and Health in the Elderly McIntosh I.B. 1992 Quay Publications. Lancaster.
3 Cossar J. Reid D. et al 1990 Cumulative review of studies o travellers J . Infect. 21 27-42
4 McIntosh I. Travel induced illness 1991 Scot. Med. 11.4.14-15
5 Source: Census, April 2001, Office for National Statistics General Register Office ,Scotland
 6 Cameron J 1991.Functions in the elderly. Ger. Med. 29-34
7 Villar P.Wiggins J et al 1991Structure and function of the ageing lung Care of the Elderly 3.129
8 Abrams W. Berror R 1990 Manual of geriatrics. Merck & Co New Jersey
9 McIntosh I B. Psychological features of travel 2008 Brit Trav Health Assoc .J. 11. 34-7

Chapter Two

Pretravel Risk Assessment

"A man is as old as his arteries." Sydenham[1].

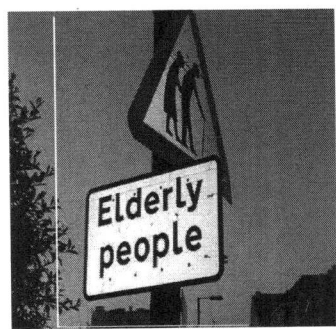

PRETRAVEL RISK ASSESSMENT

The pretravel health consultation provides opportunity to gather general and health data from potential travellers, to identify factors, which may impact on their health status while abroad and initiate measures to minimise or prevent adverse effects. Creation of a personalised database is essential. Management requires consideration of potential hazards -untoward events, which may occur- and risk, which relates to the degree of chance that an event will occur. Many factors are involved. For instance, disease hazard in a country depends not only on its presence, but other elements such as climate, sanitation, water supply, disease vectors and carriers, with level of health risk determined by personal immunity, vaccination, and exposure to infection.

Identifying the risk

Data to be acquired:	Considerations
Age and gender	Elderly, very old
Regional destination	Developing country
Season	Monsoon
Travel duration	short/ long haul
Holiday type	Visit to relatives/ city tours/ Safari/Upcountry/Adventure/Sporting
Climate	climatic extremes

Altitude	high altitude
Latitude	high/ low latitude
Transportation mode	air/ sea /land
Itinerary	touring / static
Holiday activities	sporting /adventure
Vaccination status	
Smoking status	
Current physical status	Functional ability
Psychological status	Personality. travel phobia/ confusional /anxiety state
Past medical history	
Current health status	
Pre-existing chronic disease	
Health facilities at destination.	Quality, proximity
Travel health insurance status.	Adequacy, exclusions

Those suffering from pre-existing disease suffer the further disadvantage of physical constraints relating to the condition. They are less able to compensate for the demands of a hostile environment and are more likely to succumb to travel-induced illness and disease.

Factors which influence health risk

AGE Effects

Each consultation with an elderly potential traveller should consider the impact of the ageing process on the individual. Aging organs gradually, but progressively, lose function and there is decrease in maximum functioning capacity. This often goes unnoticed by the individual as organs have a reserve ability to function beyond routine needs, but travel can bring additional physiological demands.

The heart of a 20-year-old is capable of pumping 10 times the amount that is actually needed to preserve life. After age 30, about 1% of this reserve is lost annually. With advanced years, an organ when worked harder than usual, may not be able to increase function eg. sudden *heart failure* can develop. Body stressors e.g. disease, life changes such as an energetic vacation, suddenly increased physical demands on the body from change in physical activity and exposure to high altitude can produce extra cardiac load. The effects of ageing on the heart, lungs, kidney and brain can make older world travellers more vulnerable to travel-related disease and trauma than younger people.[2]

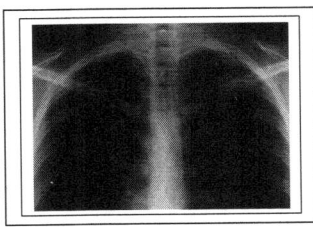

Ageing Heart

Heart functions slow down with age. The aging process reduces heart muscle strength so pumping power declines, and maximal heart rate also decreases. When the amount of blood pumped by the heart in a minute declines, systolic blood pressure tends to rise. Ageing of the heart is associated with a number of disease-independent changes associated with a reduction in function including:-

- a fall in number of myocytes and cells within the conduction tissue,
- development of cardiac fibrosis,
- reduction in calcium transport across membranes,
- lower capillary density,
- decrease in the intracellular response to Beta-adrenergic stimulation.

There is a steady increase in heart size and thickness of ventricular walls with age, with the cardiovascular system becoming more susceptible to diseases including high blood pressure and atherosclerosis. Nearly 40 % of all deaths among those 65 and older are due to heart problems.

By 80 years, men are nine times and women eleven times more likely to die of chronic heart failure than they were at age 50.[1]

The older heart—even in the very fit—is no match for a younger one during exercise or stress. During physical activity the heart must pump more blood to working muscles. In the young it increases the heart rate and squeezing harder during contractions, sends more blood with each beat. The response differs with ageing. Heart rate still rises, but not as high.

In 20 year olds, maximum rate is 190 to 200 beats per minute; by age 80, this has diminished to 145 beats, with substantial decline in the peak rate at which the older heart can beat. The force of contraction during vigorous exercise increases, but not as much in older people as in the young and cardiovascular reserve diminishes.

A 20-year-old can increase cardiac output during exercise to 3-4 times over resting levels, but an 80 year old can only muster about two times. The Frank-Starling mechanism compensates in part for this shortfall, however during vigorous exercise the older heart still pumps less blood overall because it can not beat as fast as a young heart.This adaptation helps the heart meet immediate needs of the exercising older body, but it increases heart load and forces it to work harder. Ventricles do not fully relax between beats, causing end diastolic left ventricular pressure to increase and left atrial pressure rises. This pressure increase is transmitted to lungs and as pressure rises, oxygenated blood struggles to get from lungs into the left side of heart to be pumped out to the body. The person then exhibits dyspnoea with effort.[2]

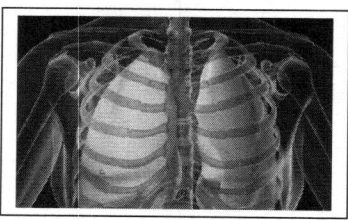

Ageing Lungs

Abnormalities occur in the aging human lung which include:-

- decreased mucociliary function,
- dilatation of airspaces,
- loss of elastic recoil,
- loss of elastin fibres,
- Diminished diffusion capacity,

These changes explain the progressive decline of pulmonary function,[3] which gradually occurs after age 20. In the absence of respiratory insults (e.g., smoking, environmental toxins, prior respiratory infections), most elderly people have sufficient respiratory reserve to avoid symptoms. Reduction of respiratory reserve with ageing however often increases the risk and severity of pulmonary infections. After age 20, the number of alveoli and lung capillaries gradually begin to decrease, although, lung volumes, airflow, diffusing capacity, and purely age-related changes of lung function do not lead to clinically significant symptoms in non-smokers. In smokers and former smokers, injury due to inflammation is superimposed on and accelerates the effects of aging, resulting in dyspnoea.

Changes in lung and chest wall compliance are primarily responsible for age-related decreases in ventilation and the corresponding decreases in gas distribution that result from collapse of small airways. After age 30, there is decrease in number and elasticity of parenchymal elastic fibres, which causes gradual loss of elastic recoil of the lungs. Airway size also decreases.

After 55 years, respiratory muscles begin to weaken, and chest wall gradually becomes stiffer (decreasing compliance). The increased outward pull of the stiffer chest wall combined with the reduced ability of the lung to pull inward result in a small increase in functional residual capacity and residual volume

Diffusing capacity peaks in people in early 20s and then declines. From middle age onward, it declines at a rate of about 17% per decade in men and at a rate of about 15% in women The loss of alveolar-capillary surface area decreases venous blood oxygenation, particularly under conditions of high pulmonary blood flow (e.g., exercise)

Partial pressure of arterial oxygen (PaO2) declines linearly with ageing (about 0.3%/year) until age 75, at which time it stabilizes at about 80 mm Hg in healthy non-smokers.[4]

Autonomic Response in ageing.

Heart rate and ventilatory responses to hypoxia and hypercapnia diminish with aging because peripheral and central chemoreceptor responses diminish. Aging also decreases neural output to respiratory muscles and lowers chest wall and lung mechanical efficiency. As a result, ventilatory response to hypoxia is reduced by 51% in healthy men aged 64 to 73 years compared with healthy men aged 22 to 30; ventilatory response to hypercapnia is reduced by 41%. After age 40, decreases in FEV1 and FVC occur due to aging itself. There are also superimposed cumulative effects of inflammatory injury from respiratory illness, smoking, and exposure to environmental toxins.[5]

Blood and circulation changes

Aging causes a reduction in total body water so there is less fluid in the bloodstream, with decreased blood volume. The number of red blood cells is reduced which contributes to fatigue. Blood vessels become less elastic with "average" blood pressure increasing from 120/70 to 150/90 mm,Hg., Blood vessels lose elasticity and respond more slowly to change in body position with resultant postural hypotension, dizziness and falls.[2]

Other systemic deterioration

Body temperature changes

Body temperature does not change significantly with advanced years, but temperature regulation, is more difficult. Loss of subcutaneous fat makes it harder to maintain body heat. Skin changes include reduced ability to sweat. Older people find it more difficult to tell when they are becoming overheated and are at greater risk from hyperthermia or heat stroke. They are also affected by dangerous drops in body temperature (hypothermia).[6]

Immunity change

There is a decline in immunity, associated with increased vulnerability to infectious agents, with several causes of immuno-senescence. The progressive atrophy of the thymus gland occurring with ageing, affects ability to generate a cell-mediated immune response. The thymus gland is where T lymphocyte ("T cell") immune cells mature. The thymus begins to atrophy and by middle age is about 15% of its maximum size at adolescence although the number of T cells does not decrease with aging, T cell function decreases, causing a weakening of the parts of the immune system controlled by these T cells.

Elderly people produce fewer helper T cells and the ones they do have are often less effective than they were earlier in life.

These changes bring slow, steady decrease in immunity after young adulthood. When the body is exposed to bacteria or micro-organisms by actual exposure or by immunization, fewer protective antibodies may be formed or they form slower. Diminution of cell-mediated immune response with age, leads to a progressive reduction in antigen- driven lymphocyte proliferation , a common deficit in elderly individuals. Antibody responses to some vaccines (eg. pneumococcal, influenza) that can decrease the risk of pneumonia decline with increased age. Cellular immunity also declines with age. Influenza immunisation and other immunisations may be less effective and protection may not last as long as expected. The immune system also becomes less able to detect foreign particles and infection risk is greater.

Other factors related to ageing also increase the risk of infections such as sensation and skin change , which increase the risk of injury and permit bacterial skin entry . Ageing also affects inflammation – an immune response – and wound healing which proceeds more slowly.[7]

Ageing Kidney

- decline in glomerular filtration rate,
- decreased urinary concentration
- decrease in diluting ability,
- diminished urinary acidification,
- impaired potassium clearance.
- proneness to drug toxicity,
- fluid and electrolyte imbalance, especially when dehydrated.

Kidneys have a built-in extra capacity. However, decreased efficiency occurs when they are under increased workload from illness, medications, and dehydration. Renal changes may affect ability to concentrate urine and hold onto water with response to fluids and electrolyte intake slowed. Dehydration can occur more readily in older people who frequently have less sense of thirst. The bladder wall changes with age with elastic tissue replaced by tough fibrous tissue, and the organ becomes less distensible.[8,9,10] Muscles weaken, and the bladder may not empty completely when urinating with resultant continence problems [10]

Ageing skin:

Thinning occurs as the rate of cell production slows in the epidermis. The dermis may also become thinner, more 'papery'. Less elastin fibres are produced causing sagging and drooping. Melanocytes tend to increase in certain areas, like backs of hands, forming age or liver spots. Older skin has fewer sweat and oil glands, with reduced ability to sweat. Loss of subcutaneous fat makes it harder to maintain body heat. Older people also find it more difficult to tell when they are becoming overheated.

Ageing Brain:

As people get older, there is a decrease in brain weight and brain volume, widening of the grooves on the surface of the brain and enlargement of the ventricular system, probably due to loss of cells surrounding the ventricles Decrease in brain weight and brain volume are probably due to loss of neurons and extra cellular fluid. A person may have a 20% reduction in brain weight between the ages of forty -five and eighty -five and loss of thirty to fifty thousand neurons a day from the brain and nervous system with ageing.

Two thirds of old people eventually experience some significant loss of mental lucidity and independence as a result of aging. Individuals 60 years and older, often experience cognitive decline including:-

- impairment in memory,
- loss of concentration,
- decreased clarity of thought,
- impairment in focus and judgment.

The way the brain processes information is slowed, affecting the rate that people can put new information into permanent memory, especially factual information. With aging, delayed recall occurs— not being able to remember a familiar name or word — and it becomes harder to pay attention to more than one thing at a time. Common factors that impair normal memory function are, stress, alcohol use, lack of sleep, all elements associated with international travel.[6]

Bone changes:

In early life, a careful balance exists between bone formation by osteoblasts and bone resorption by osteoclasts. With aging, the process of coupled bone formation is affected by the reduction of osteoblast differentiation, activity, and life span, which is further, potentiated in the per-menopausal years with hormone deprivation and increased osteoclast activity. Resultant osteoporosis can bring fracture from minor falls.[11]

Sensorial change:

At age 70, 30% people have impairment of vision and hearing. At 81 years, 6% have low vision and moderate to severe hearing loss, and one-tenth normal vision and hearing. At 88 years, 8-13% have low vision and moderate to severe hearing loss and no men and less than one-tenth of women have normal vision and hearing.[12]

Sight:

Loss of accommodation and focussing.The extent the pupil can dilate decreases with age. The light adapted eye at 20 years gets 6 times greater light to eye than an 80 year old. The 20 year old, dark-adapted eye gets 16 times greater light to retina than an 80 year old. There is an age related delay in dark adaptation. Failing visual acuity with advancing years creates difficulties in reading instructions and locomotion with old particularly vulnerable in low light situations.[12]

Hearing:

Older people develop presbyacusis, with as many as half over 75 having hearing loss. As a person ages, cochlear hair cells may become damaged. This results in a high-frequency hearing loss that can start as early as middle age, with males more affected over 40 years old. The middle ear also ages, going through physical changes that make it more difficult for a person to discriminate sound. Hearing loss is most pronounced at higher frequencies for both sexes. Loss of auditory acuity makes for difficulty hearing public address systems[13]

Environmental stress and ageing.

Stress – the physical or psychological condition elicited by a situation- can be perceived as an external danger, hazard, threat or challenge. It places demands on the person who responds with coping mechanisms and adaptation.[14]

Relocation and international travel are stressors. Elderly people with more rigid thought processes can be slow to adapt and coping strategies may be less confrontational. They may be less likely to 'stand up for their rights' and have slower reaction times in emergency situations.[15,16,17]

The effects of existing disease

Illness, or recent surgery, can further weaken the immune system, making the body more susceptible to subsequent infections. Diabetes, more prevalent with age, can lead to decreased immunity. Reductions in ventilatory response increase the risks of developing hypoxia and hypercapnia if elderly people acquire disorders that produce low O2 levels (e.g., pneumonia, COPD, obstructive sleep apnoea

Chronically low oxygen levels in the elderly, reduce tolerance to illness, decreased exercise tolerance, abnormal breathing patterns including apnoea, increased risk of lung infections such as pneumonia, or bronchitis and diseases caused by tobacco damage such as emphysema. Additional factors for cardiovascular decline in function are disease insults such as diabetes, hypertension, hyperlipidaemia and the habit of smoking.[7]

Aging increases the risk for urinary disorders including acute and chronic renal failure. Bladder infections and other urinary tract infections are more common in seniors, in part, related to incomplete bladder emptying. Urinary retention is more common as is urinary incontinence. The aging kidney is constantly exposed to the effects of a variety of potential toxic processes, i.e., drugs and chronic illnesses including hypertension, diabetes, and atherosclerotic disease.[8] Renal changes that occur with aging also consist of impairment in the ability to concentrate urine and to conserve sodium and water. These physiological changes increase the risks of volume depletion and prerenal type of acute renal failure.viii In men, the urethra may become blocked by an enlarged prostate gland. In women, weakened muscles can allow the bladder or vagina to prolapse, also causing blockage and urinary difficulties. With often-restricted access to toilets in world travel these are serious considerations for older travellers.8.9.10

Medication

Long term medication can also add to health risk with potential effect on prophylaxis and travel related health threats and failed compliance which is common in travellers.

Age effects on bodily function which can increase the risks of world travel

Decreased heart capacity decreases ability to cope with travel related stresses such dehydration, high altitude or physical exertion.

- Decreased lung capacity means less reserve to deal with reduced oxygen at altitude or from chest infection.
- Weakened immune system makes infection more likely
- Deteriorating kidney function increases likelihood that dehydration will lead to kidney failure and diminishes ability for kidneys to cope with salt loss when diarrhoea occurs
- Deteriorating brain function can cause confusion in stressful situations and some elderly people find difficulty in coping with new situations and have a lower anxiety threshold
- Decline in visual and auditory senses can cause accidents or failure to see or hear public announcements in airports , rail stations and on ships.
- Poor balance and slow reaction time can increase risk of fall, and make walking more perilous
- Poorer circulation and wound healing results in slower healing of scratches, bites and injuries.
- Thinning bones from osteoporosis increase the risk of fractures with falls.
- Reduced stomach acid increases risk from food poisoning and contaminated food and water 6

Increased vulnerability during travel due to:

- high temperatures and heat stroke
- environmental extremes
- deep vein thrombosis
- hypothermia
- effects of low oxygen
- fatigue and exhaustion

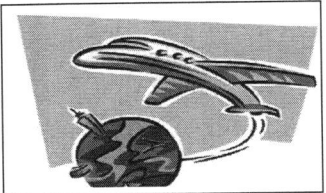

FACTORS AFFECTING ALL TRAVELLERS

Destination

Certain regions of the world, primarily developing countries present higher health risk due to the risk of infection and road traffic accident.

Season

Travel off the tourist season, in the monsoon or in extreme heat or cold can be hazardous for the traveller

Transportation

Air travel over 8 hours duration and prolonged coach and car travel can create a traveller's thrombosis risk

Holiday type. Visitors to friends and relatives in Africa and Asia can be at higher risk of infection as they assume immunity and do not acquire appropriate vaccinations

Climate Extremes of heat or cold can result in travellers suffering heat stroke, dehydration, hyperthermia and hypothermia

Local medical facilities. In emergency local medical and nursing aid may be substandard, inadequate and distant with prolonged evacuation to the disadvantage of the ill or injured traveller

Assessment and management Planning

Management Plan.

1. Identify health hazards using a questionnaire

2 Analyse the risk

3 Advise patients of health hazards in the proposed

   travel itinerary

4 Advise on factors, which can be altered to decrease risk

5 Negotiate a management plan and programme with the client.

6 Provide adequate prophylaxis and vaccination

7 Provide appropriate advice regarding precautions to be taken

   en route, at the destination and on return

8 Counsel on appropriate changes in drug medication e.g. with

diabetes, and how to deal with alterations in

circadian rhythm

9 Advise about minimising the effects of pre-existing disease

during travel and on holiday

10 Provide appropriate certificates and referral letters

11 Complete of certificates required by transport authorities,or tour operators

12 Advise clients on sources of useful information booklets, websites

13 Provide clinical valuation for the high risk, very frail old and for those with pre-existing disease which may exclude them from travel. Much of the assessment in these procedures can be carried out by members of the Care Team; ie practice or travel clinic nurse.[8]

Data acquisition

Acquisition of the data from one to one consultation, or from a questionnaire presented to the patient on arrival at the pretravel interview, will provide the necessary information for the health professional to make an informed risk assessment of the health hazards likely to confront the person on international travel. Analysis of data will identify the traveller at higher risk and permit creation of a customised management plan to minimise or negate potential challenge to health. The client can be apprised of risks, encouraged to recognise them and advised on appropriate prophylaxis and prevention. Creation of a customised management plan for the individual, to minimise risk of global travel is recommended:

Risk appraisal.

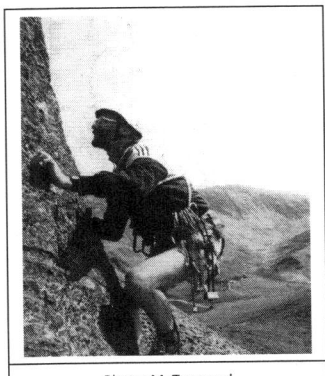

Photo: M. Townend

Advanced age makes world travellers more vulnerable to trauma and infection but other key factors affecting a sojourn abroad must be considered .It can help to sort travellers into low, medium and high-risk categories with a scoring tool based on the questionnaire.[ii]Destinations in developing countries, the tropics, environmental and latititudinal extremes and more distant countries in the former eastern bloc, may present high risk. Travel in the monsoon season, on safari, up-country and for adventure and sport are also likely to be riskier health undertakings. Prolonged travel by air or coach can present health hazard and people visiting family and friends often risk disease by failing to take appropriate vaccinations. Smokers, the unvaccinated and those with predisposing or chronic disease have to be regarded as potentially higher risk travellers.

A risk-scoring tool[18]			
	low	medium	high
Age – 65-74	*		
75-84		*	
85+			*
Risk Scoring Tool	low	medium	high
Destination - Northern Europe, Canada, America, Australia, New Zealand	*		
Eastern Europe, Former Soviet bloc, Mediterranean littoral		*	
Tropics, SE Asia , India, Africa. Developing countries			*
Season - favourable	*		
monsoon, out of season		*	
Transportation-air ,long-haul,		*	
Sea, land	*		
Climate/ - moderate, low altitude	*		
environment extreme, high altitude			*
Smoking status – non smoker	*	*	

	low	medium	high
smoker			
Physiological function-*functional, visual, hearing, continence defect*		*	
Psychological state-*travel phobia, anxiety/ confusional state*		*	
Medical status-*current illness*, *pre-existing and chronic illness*, **terminal** *illness*		*	
Medications *-multiple*		*	
	low	*medium*	*high*
Predisposition to severe motion sickness		*	
Vaccination status *– unprotected, immuno-suppressed*			*
Medical facilities at destination *poor, distant*			*
RISK Scoring tool	*low*	*medium*	*high*
Travel insurance *–absent, inadequate*		*	
Recent stroke, myocardial infarction, insulin dependent diabetic, COAD <50%			*

Summating the score in predominantly medium and high risk categories will help to identify those who should have a comprehensive health screen before departure 18

Infection risk

The risk of the traveller succumbing to infection while overseas has to be gauged. This is an important determinant of advice and vaccination to be proffered.xiv Figure one provides a rough guide to risk per month of travel

Figure 1
Risk per month of travel (after Steffen *et al*, 1997)

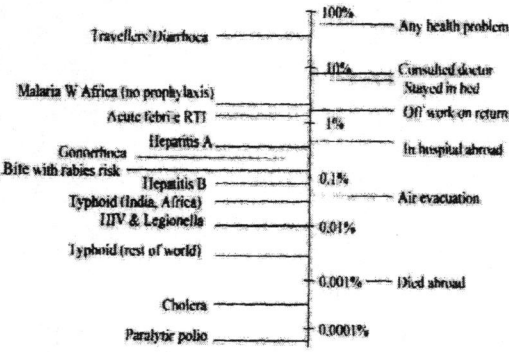

This is a logarithmic chart. Each graduation represents a 10-fold difference in risk. 100% would imply that all travellers would be likely to develop the problem, 1% that 1 in 100 travellers would be likely to develop it and 0.0001 that 1 in 1 million would be likely to develop it.

19

Summary

Increased vulnerability in the old is due to;-

- Increased infection risk
- Decreased ability to fight diseases
- Slowed wound healing
- Change in gait
- Imbalance
- Poor temperature control
- Decreased immunity
- Increased health risk with heavy exercise, high altitude, environmental extremes, physical and psychological stress.
- Renal changes
- Decreased cardiovascular efficiency
- Ventilatory changes
- Skin thinning
- Cognitive impairment
- Less ability to cope with psychological stressors
- Pre-existing illness.
- Medications.[19]

References

1 Sydenham, T. English Physician, 1624-1689.
2 Roffe C. Ageing of the heart. 1998. Br. J. Biomed Sci. 55.2, 136-48.
3 Signola, AM. Bousquet J The Ageing Lung 2001.Current Allergy Reports, 1:1–2Current Science Inc.
4 Cameron J 1991.Functions in the elderly. Ger. Med. 29-34.
5 Villar P.Wiggins J et al 1991 Structure and function of the ageing lung. Care of the Elderly 3.129.
6 Abrams W Berror R 1990 Manual of geriatrics. Merck & Co New Jersey.
7 Overstall PW in Medicine. 1994 Ed. Souhami R. Moxham J Churchill Livingstone. Edinburgh.
8 Zhou XJ. Saxena R.Liu Z.et al Renal senescence in 2008:progress and challenges. Int.Urol. Nephrol 2008;40(3):823-39. E pub 2008.
9 Muhlberg W Platt D. Age dependent changes of the kidneys,pharmacological implications. Gerontology 1999.
10 Meyer BR. Bellucci A. Renal function in the elderly. Cardiol Clin.1986 4(2) 227-34.
11 Chan G, Duque G. Age-Related Bone Loss: Old Bone, New Facts. Internat. J.Exptl.Clin Behave and Tech Gerontology. 2002 48.2.
12 Bergman B. Rosenhall U. Vision and hearing in old age Scand.Audiol.2001;3:255-63.
13 Pedersen K. Rosenhall U.Muller M Changes in pure tone thresh holds. Audiology 1989;28(4):194-204.
14 Simonton KN Presbycusis, hearing loss of old age Geriatrics.1955 10.7.337-8
15 Costa P.McRae A. Ageing Stress and Health 1990 Wiley. Chichester.
16 McIntosh I. Power K. et al Prevalence, and intensity of travel related stressors J. Trav. Med. 1996 3.2.96-102
17 McIntosh I. Power K. et al Anxiety and health problems related to air travel J. Trav. Med. 1998. 5.198-204
18 McIntosh I. Travel and health in the elderly - A medical handbook 1992 Quay Publishing Lancaster.
19 Townend M. Risk assessment .Brit. Trav. Health. Assoc J.2008.12

Iain B.McIntosh

Chapter 3

Travel related illness and trauma.

Infection risk and avoidance

As to diseases ,make a habit of two things – to help or at least do no harm. Hippocrates.

All travellers are exposed to a range of health risks during a trip overseas. Health professionals need to be aware of these and how to prevent them if best advice is to be provided to clients.

Older travellers may be more vulnerable to these risks and if they are affected may be more adversely disturbed. Lowered immunity makes it more likely they may become infected and secondary effects of infection such as fever, dehydration and electrolyte imbalance can prove a greater health threat than in younger people. They are at greater risk of having a road traffic accident while abroad. The effects of trauma with fracture, disability and slower healing may have greater impact on seniors.

Risk can be divided into two categories and the actual risk to the individual is dependent upon prevalence of the condition at destination or en route Travel destination is associated with the probability of the diagnosis of certain diseases. Significant trends are based on regional differences:

Infectious-health risk

- Dengue
- Diphtheria
- Hepatitis A,B,C,D,E
- HIV and sexually transmitted infections
- Influenza
- Japanese encephalitis
- Legionnaires' disease
- Leishmaniasis
- Leptospirosis
- Lyme disease
- Malaria
- Meningococcal meningitis
- Poliomyelitis
- Rabies
- Rickettsial disease
- Schistosomiasis
- Tetanus
- Tick-borne encephalitis
- Traveller's diarrhoea

Infections –health risk contd.
- Trypanosomiasis
- Tuberculosis
- Typhoid and paratyphoid
- West Nile virus
- Yellow fever

Non-infectious environmental health risk
- Altitude illness
- Insect and animal bite
- Sun protection
- Accident
- Travel related deep vein thrombosis

It is estimated that 5% of travel related infectious disease is vaccine preventable.[1]

In returning travellers:-

- fever with only generalized symptoms occurs disproportionately among those returning from sub-Saharan Africa or Southeast Asia,
- acute diarrhoea occurs most frequently in those returning from south central Asia,
- dermatological problems primarily present in those returning from Caribbean area, Central or South America
- malaria is one of the three most frequent causes of systemic fever-related illness among travellers from every region,
- travellers from every region except sub-Saharan Africa and Central America have confirmed or probable dengue more frequently than malaria
- Travellers from all regions except Southeast Asia presented with parasite-induced diarrhoea more often than with bacterial diarrhoea.

Travel related illness

The risk for infections is high during travel and visits to many developing countries.[2] However, disease causes just 9% of deaths. To determine the incidence of travel-related illness in a typical urban population in Scotland, 1568 patients, presenting within a 1-year period at a medical practice were studied and morbidity rates investigated. 42% of travellers became ill while abroad, with 48% of ill travellers returning to consult their family doctor. Travellers to Africa and Asia were shown to have the highest rates of illness .[3]People who consulted a doctor were likely to be older, in poorer health and taking regular medication, FGI is common.[4]

In a sample of ill-returned travellers .The male-to-female ratio was 1.6 Most patients (70.9%) were returning from sub-Saharan Africa. the median time from return of travel to hospitalization was 13 days (IQR, 7-21). Malaria was the most frequent diagnosis (49.1%), which was especially encountered in patients returning from sub-Saharan Africa (95.6%), without adequate chemoprophylaxis (78.2%) [5]

Adventure travel places travellers at added health risk from environmental hazards, which are important causes of morbidity and potential mortality among travellers. Injuries are common among adventure travellers (6.1%)[6,7]

Travellers Diarrhoea

Traveller's diarrhoea is the number one problem in international tourism in terms of frequency, personal and economic impact.[5] It can have deleterious effects on aged tourists who succumb to the infection if there is marked fluid loss with electrolyte imbalance. That and the associated dehydration may increase the likelihood of angina, arrythmias including atrial fibrillation, myocardial and cerebral infarction. If elderly adventurous travellers do become ill from diarrhoea while overseas, delay in access to supportive medical and nursing services may compound the health problem. Elderly travellers are more likely to acquire gastrointestinal infection than younger people due to lower immunity, and are less able to combat the infection. Decreased renal function make also more difficult for them to maintain water and electrolyte balance. Vomiting and diarrhoea with fluid and electrolyte imbalance may also have an impact on chronic disorder such as diabetes mellitus and routine medications may be disturbed in the ill.[3]

Estimates suggest 50,000 travellers a day suffer from traveller's diarrhoea in high-risk countries. Fortunately mortality due to traveller's diarrhoea is uncommon but 1% of people are ill enough to require hospital admission.[8,9] Risk is associated with destination, length of stay and dependent upon ingestion of contaminated food or water which is responsible for most cases with the commonest cause due to bacteria. Countries can be identifies as low-, medium and high-risk with risk altering seasonally in temperate climates. It has been estimated that 30-50% of travellers will develop traveller's diarrhoea during a 1- to 2-week stay in high-risk areas.[10] People who consulted a doctor were likely to be older, in poorer health and taking regular medication.

Risk areas for transmission of travellers diarrhoea:-

Low-risk
North America, Australia, New Zealand, Japan, Northwest Europe.

Medium risk
Eastern Europe and former eastern bloc countries, South Africa, Caribbean area

High-risk
Middle East, SE Asia but not Singapore, Africa –north and central Africa, South America

Traveller's diarrhoea can be debilitating and dangerous for older individuals as they can become dehydrated and enter in to electrolyte imbalance. 30-50% of travellers to high-risk areas become ill during a 1-2 week visit, approximately 50,000 cases of traveller's diarrhoea occur each day.[9] Microorganisms responsible for traveller's diarrhoea include:-

Bacteria
Enterotoxigenic *E. coli* (ETEC):
Enteroaggregative *E. coli* (EAEC):
***Campylobacter jejuni*:**

Bacteria contd
Salmonella spp.
10% of cases of traveller's diarrhoea is caused by Protozoan parasites The most common parasites responsible for traveler's diarrhoea include:
Parasites
Giardia lamblia:
Cryptosporidium parvum:
Cyclospora cayetensis:
Giardia lamblia,).
Entamoeba histolytica:.
Enteric viral infections are responsible for only 5-10% of cases of traveller's diarrhoea, illness can be debilitating. Norovirus and rotavirus are responsible for most cases of enteric viral infection.

Malaria
Malaria is not endemic in the uk, but nearly 2000 cases occur annually in travellers returning to the uk from malaria-endemic countries. Malaria is a preventable, disease transmitted by the the female *anopheles* mosquito.The types that affect humans are *plasmodium falciparum* (causing most deaths), *vivax,* *ovale,* and *malariae* resulting in one million deaths per year world wide.the disease mainly occurs in Africa, Asia ,South and Central america, , and the Middle east. One million deaths from malaria occur worldwide each year.

Analysis of people travelling abroad in2007showed 18% were in people visiting friends and relatives(vfr) with a significant number of them travelling to countries with a high prevalence of malaria, typhoid, paratyphoid and hepatitis A, and India, Pakistan and Bangladesh in particular. Many did not seek travel health advice before the trip and the majority did not take malaria prophylaxis. Many of these vfrs. are first generation immigrants returning to their former homeland and those in the first wave of post war immigration are now of senior years. They assume they have an immunity from their previous residence abroad but this is illusory and they need anti malarial and other protection.[11]

Case History

A couple in their mid–seventies were travelling in a group on a conventional tourist trip along the old Silk Road to Samarkand. They both unwisely enjoyed an ice cream from a roadside vendor in Tashkent. Through the next night the wife became ill with vomiting, profuse diarrhoea, fever and prostration. The hospital doctor arranged admission to the local infectious disease unit and for the husband to remain in the hotel until the return of the group a week later.
The wife was treated with magnesium trisilicate and fluids in the district hospital which had few resources. She slowly returned to health. The husband was left isolated, in his own care, in an environment with no English speakers He soon fell ill with travellers' diarrhoea. The local water supply was contaminated and he did not replace his fluid loss as bottled water was expensive. At the end of the week when the main party returned, he was found to be ill, confused, extremely dehydrated and suffering watery diarrhoea. Hospitalised, he received the same treatment as the wife and made a partial recovery. Flown back to the UK. with an accompanying nurse,he was readmitted to hospital in Britain in gross electrolyte imbalance and renal failure and died shortly afterwards. His death was untimely, travel related, potentially avoidable and the outcome not inevitable if treatment had been prompt and adequate.

Accidents

Travellers often suffer a road traffic accident at the start or end of their travels while travelling to airport or port. The UK national estimate for accidents while travelling and touring was 480,66 in 2007. Statistics show that the chance of being involved in a car accident however in mainland Europe doubles, and it almost triples in Greece and Portugal.[11]

Accidents cause 20% of all deaths among overseas travellers – the second most common cause after heart disease (68%).
Accidents can occur through, road accidents, personal violence, accidental injury

Road accidents

Accidents in vehicles or on the road are one of the riskiest aspects of travel abroad.

Accidental injury

In the UK there are 2 million accidents and 6,000 deaths each year in the home. Unfamiliar surroundings in a foreign environment will increase these risks.
Falls are a common cause of injury and are often associated with alcohol. They are particularly likely in older adults, due to poor vision, imbalance and postural hypotension
Walking barefoot or in sandals increases the risk of falls and foot injuries.

Personal violence

Most violence occurs through muggings or theft.

Accidents are far more of a risk abroad than less likely sources of danger, such as terrorism or exotic diseases, which travellers often fear.

Accidents are a serious travel related risk accounting for about 25% of all deaths of travellers while abroad[13,14]Accidents kill and injure many travellers with 28% of accidental deaths due to road traffic tragedies. Developing countries have 20 times more traffic accidents per road miles than developed countries. Particularly high risk road activities are travelling in unsafe vehicles, by motor scooter or over-crowded bus. [15] Older drivers have a higher crash risk per mile driven than other adults. The "risk" of dying in a crash is more likely, attributable to the frailty of older drivers than the risks associated with the functional limitations that accompany aging. Research literature indicates that older drivers are not a risk to other road user age groups but primarily to themselves. It is the older driver and their vehicle occupants who are at higher risk of dying when in a crash.[16]

Altitude Illness

High altitude-above 5,000 metres- with decreasing partial pressure of oxygen, can expose the traveller to acute mountain sickness. This can be related to the strenuous individual climbing too fast, too high and too far on a day of travel in high mountains. Older people are perhaps less likely than the young to exhibit this behaviour and are no more likely than other adults to succumb to the condition. However, lungs and heart have not the performance of younger climbers and lower pO_2 can push older people into cardiac and respiratory failure, with those with underlying cardio/pulmonary disease at greatest risk. [7]The majority of elderly people exposed to high altitude will be travelling to destinations in South America where cities like La Paz and Cusco have airports 4,000 metres above sea level. Many people arriving here are unaware of the risk until they find themselves with laboured breathing and anoxia or angina in the rarified atmosphere.

Pretravel Preparation

In anticipation of distant foreign travel the elderly person should consider a travel health consultation and the docor/nurse and the individual should appraise the health risk and consider prevention and protection. The traveller should seek appropriate vaccination and malaria prophylaxis. The need for mechanical protection against mosquito bites has to be emphasised and repellents should be used in conjunction with prophylactic medication.[17]

Gp and commercial travel health clinic staff can then provide a customised action plan. Travel health clinics significantly reduce the morbidity of illness for travellers and the burden on general practices can be reduced with pretravel advice and prophylaxis Travel clinic attendees are more likely to be travelling to high-risk destinations, but are better prepared, experiencing a significantly lower rate of illness during travel (22%). Clinic attendees are also less likely to consult their doctor regarding travel related dullness on return home.[6]

Cochrane Collaboration database of systematic reviews and meta-analyses was searched for studies relevant to family physicians and there are no randomised control trials on preventing accidents and abroad.

Patient Information Leaflets

Avoidance of Injuries from 'natural hazards'.

- Foot injuries in those unfamiliar with wearing sandals or when going barefoot are common.Sensible footwear should be worn.
- Sea creatures (e.g. fish, eels, mollusks) and caterpillars may be unexpectedly venomous causing rashes or more serious illnesses.Wear protective footwear when entering unfamiliar water.
- Dogs and cats in many countries run wild, are often hungry and may respond aggressively when approached. Avoid handling them.
- Do some homework and be aware of where the nearest emergency facilities are situated

Avoiding Road accidents

- Be aware driving custom may be on the opposite side of the road to UK.
- Reliable cars should be used. Examine the car carefully and ensure it is roadworthy, has seat belts and use them. Avoid driving in poor light and at night.
- Strictly observe speed limits, traffic lights and other road signs
- Never drink and drive.
- Be very careful on potholed and non-sealed gravel roads which can become corrugated.
- Avoid overcrowded buses.

- Hiring scooters and motor bicycles is risky. Ensure that safety helmets are used

Ensuring Personal Safety (mugging, theft, violence)

- Most authorities say that travellers should not resist if mugged. It is better to lose valuables than be injured or worse

Prevention of diarrhoea

The Cochrane Collaboration database of systematic reviews for preventing diarrhoea confirms that randomised control trials demonstrate that bismuth subsalicylate, doxycycline, ciprofloxacin, and trimethoprim-sulfamethoxazole are useful prophylactics.[18]Where food and water is concerned, 'boil,cook, peel or avoid it' is good advice. The second generation prebiotic food supplement B-GOS taken immediately prior to and during travel, may be of value in preventing or diminishing the impact of travel related diarrhoea.[19]

Prevention of malaria

The Advisory Committee on Malaria Prevention for UK Travellers (ACMP) has produced guidelines of essential information on malaria prevention for healthcare workers who advise travellers, entitled: Guidelines for Malaria Prevention in Travellers from the United Kingdom The risks of malaria need to be balanced against the risks of the preventive measures, The **ABCD** approach to prevention recognises four points essential to minimise the risk of infection.[20,12]

- **A**wareness: know about the risk of malaria
- **B**ites by mosquitoes: prevent or avoid
- **C**ompliance with appropriate chemoprophylaxis
- **D**iagnose breakthrough malaria swiftly and obtain treatment promptly

Guidelines now give greater emphasis to the importance of balancing the risk of malaria and the risk of adverse reactions to antimalarials. This depends upon:

- place to be visited
- duration of the visit
- degree of exposure
- level of drug resistance
- type of traveller

All these factors affect the risk of malaria. Most adverse reactions to antimalarials occur within the first few doses, but the cumulative risk of contracting malaria is proportional to the length of stay in a malarious area. The longer the stay, the more important it is to implement a regimen with a high protective efficacy.[12]

Prevention of altitude sickness

Use of acetazolamide as a prophylactic should be considered. The risk, benefit of the prescription has to be considered if the person has concomitant disease and is on routine medication.eg diuretic use.[21]

Information sources.
National Travel Health Network and Centre (NaTHNaC): 020 7380 9234
Glasgow, SCIEH for Travax users only, 2-4pm: 0141 300 1130
Birmingham Heartlands Hospital (Infectious Disease Unit): 0121 424 0357
Liverpool School of Tropical Medicine: 0151 708 9393
London, Northwick Park Hospital: 020 8869 28

References

1 Nathnac. Vaccine preventable illness 2007 report .London

2 Wilson E. Hospitalisation for Travel-Related Illness. Journal Watch Infectious Diseases July 8, 2005

3 McIntosh I. Elderly travellers and fitness to travel in travel Medicine and migrant health. Ed. LockieC. Walker E. et al 2000 Churchhill livingstone. London

4 Evans R. Thomas A.Howard J. Domestic and travel-related food borne gastrointestinal illness in a population health survey. 2006 Epidemiology and Infection 134:4:686-693

5 Leroy H. Arvieux C et al A retrospective study of 230 consecutive patients hospitalised for travel related illness. Eur.J. Clin. Microbiol.Infect. Disease. 2008 (11) 1137-40

6. Reed JM. McIntosh I.B Power K Travel Illness and the Family Practitioner: A Retrospective Assessment of Travel-Induced Illness in General Practice and the Effect of a Travel Illness Clinic. ....J.Trav. Med 1. 192 – 198.

7 Boggild AK,Costiniuk C, Kain KC, Pandey P. Environmental hazards in Nepal: altitude illness, environmental posures, injuries, and bites in travellers and expatriates. J Travel Med. 2007 Nov-Dec;14(6):361-8

8 Peltola HP. Gorbach LS Travellers diarrhoea in Textbook of travellers health .ed. Dupont. Steffen 1997 Decker. Canada

9 Zeichner LO Ericson CD Travellers diarrhoea in Principles and practice of travel medicine. 2001 ed. Zuckerman Wiley Chichester. Office Nat Stats. Internat. passenger survey 2007/8)

10 The Centers for Disease Control and Prevention (CDC) 2007 report.Atlanta

11 Office Nat.Stats.Internat. Passenger Survey. 2007/8 london

12 Health Protection Agency.Foreign travel associated illness –a focus on those visiting friends and relatives- 2008.London

13 Paisao MT. Cossar J. Read D. Mortality amongst overseas travellers from Scotland First Internat Cong Trav. Med. 1988 London

14 Hargarten S Baker T Guptil K Fatalities of American Travellers Proceedings. First Internat Conf Trav. Med. 1988 London

15 Eberhard J Older drivers. 2008 Traffic Inj. Prev Aug. 9 284-90

16 Petridou E Askitopolou H et al epidemiology of road accidents during pleasure travelling Accid. Anal. Prev. 1997 687-93

17 Thomas RE preparing patients to travel abroad safely 2000.Can.Fam. Physician 46 1634-8

18 *The Cochrane Database of Systematic Reviews* and *The Cochrane Library* 2003 London

19. Drakoularakou A, Tzortzis G, Rastall RA et al. A double-blind, placebo-controlled, randomized human study assessing the capacity of a novel galacto-oligosaccharide mixture in reducing travellers' diarrhoea. Eur J Clin Nutr 2009; 1-7.

20.The Advisory Committee on Malaria Prevention for UK Travellers (ACMP) Public Health Lab. Service 2008

21.Green A. Kerr A. McIntosh I. 1981 Acetazolamide in prevention of acute mountain sickness. Brit. Med. J. 283 .11

Iain B. McIntosh

Chapter 4

Air travel and Associated illness in Older Passengers

' It is not where or when you arrive, it is taking the journey that counts'.

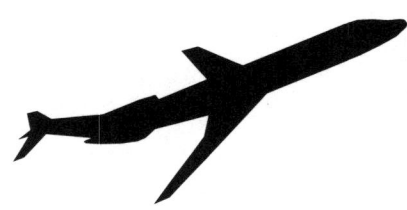

About 2 billion people travel aboard scheduled aircraft annually. 1 One in five international air journeys originates from Britain and traffic flow through British airports involves about 150 million passengers each year.2 A substantial number of them are senior citizens. They and health-care providers should be aware of potential health risks associated with air travel. Environmental and physiological changes occurring during routine commercial flights can lead to mild hypoxia and gas expansion, which can exacerbate chronic medical conditions and precipitate acute in-flight medical occurrences. The latter are increasing in frequency. With ageing of national populations, a growing number of individuals are elderly and suffering from pre-existing medical conditions. Venous thromboembolism, cosmic-radiation exposure, jet lag, cabin-air quality and psychological stress are health-care issues associated with air travel to which they are vulnerable.

Air transport is the favoured long-haul mode for protracted travel. Up to 5% of airline passengers suffer from chronic illness, with many of these elderly people given invalid passenger status. As individuals are responsible for reporting incapacity to air carriers, this may be an underestimate. 95% of individuals with health problems who have to travel by air, desire more medical advice from their physicians about its effects.3

Many older passengers instigate mid-air emergencies. About 72 people, many of advanced years, die annually while air-borne, with sudden cardiac crisis the cause of death in one group studied. Only 34% of these individuals had reported health problems prior to travel.4 Air carriers are not obliged to report in-flight medical events, but limited data report an incidence of 1 in 10,000–40,000 passengers, suggesting about 50–100 in-flight medical events per day, with United States airlines.5

In 1989/90 British Airways carried 17 million people and recorded 1328 medical incidents to airborne passengers, a gross attack rate of 1:13,000. The ratio narrowed to 1:350 of passengers, many of whom were old and infirm, who notified themselves as less than fit beforehand .The same airline reported 31, 200 medical incidents aboard their aircraft during 2007, with 3000 being deemed serious.6 Most in-flight medical events are however minor in severity[7.] The effects of pre-existing disease resulting in chronic pulmonary, cardiac, renal, hepatic and physical dysfunction can place the old at higher risk from physiological and

physical stressors inseparable from modern air travel. The air traveller faces three main problems from:-
* pressure of the air in the aircraft cabin,
* amount of oxygen in the air
* quality of air.
The first two are related. Although modern aircraft are pressurised they are not pressurised to sea level pressure but to about two thirds of sea level pressure: equivalent to the atmospheric pressure on the summit of a 2,700m.mountain. This has two consequences.
* The concentration of oxygen remains unchanged, so the actual partial pressure of oxygen must also be reduced to about two thirds of sea level.
* The reduced pressure causes gases to expand by about 30% - according to Boyle's law
.

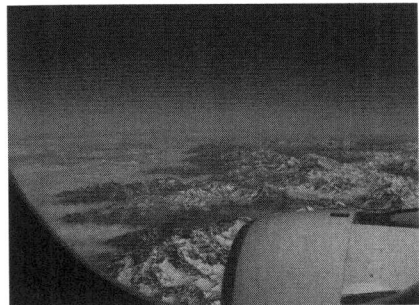

Cabin air at altitude
Tolerance to thin air experienced at altitude may be poor in passengers
suffering from chronic illness such as hypercapnia, which is associated with severe anaemia, active cerebrovascular and cardiovascular disease. Cardiac, neurological and respiratory complaints are the most serious in-flight medical events, with cardiac and neurological complaints accounting for most diversions. Passengers aged over 70 years have highest rates of in-flight medical events,[8] Individuals may cope in day to day living at ground level but exhibit fatigue, cardiac arrhythmia or vague symptoms due to anoxia, when exposed to moderate degrees of high altitude, as occurs in high flying aircraft.
Regulatory authorities require compensated cabin altitude not to exceed 2438 m. [1.9.] Healthy passengers tolerate the hypoxaemia induced by the lower than normal oxygen pressure. The arterial PO2 drops to about 8 kPa (two thirds of normal) but the shape of the oxyhaemoglobin dissociation curve ensures that saturation only falls by 5 - 6%. In passengers with respiratory disease however the changes can be more challenging. Many passengers with pre-existing cardiac, pulmonary, and haematological conditions have a reduced baseline PaO2, so reduced cabin pressure leads to further reduction of oxygen saturation, which lowers further with increasing flight times [8,9]. However, in adult volunteers simulating 20-hour flight conditions, frequency of reported complaints ie. fatigue, headache, light-headedness and nausea

increased with increasing altitude. Symptoms peaked at 2438 m, with most symptoms apparent after 3–9 hours of exposure.[10]

Cabin pressurisation to 2438 m reduces atmospheric pressure of the cabin, resulting in a concomitant decrease of arterial oxygen partial pressure (PaO2) from 95 mm Hg to60 mm Hg.[11]The decreased oxygen saturation can exacerbate medical conditions.[11,12,13,14] 18% of passengers with chronic obstructive pulmonary disease have at least mild respiratory distress during a flight. Continuous supplemental oxygen should be provided for all passengers whose saturation will fall below 85% (or P02 below 6.2 kPa) when exposed to maximum permitted altitude.[13] New aircraft, such as the Airbus A380 and Boeing 787, are designed to operate at cabin altitude of 1829 m. which should reduce hypoxic effects, but older aircraft are likely to fly around the world for decades to come.

Adverse effects of air travel

Commercial flights usually cruise at altitudes of 7010–12 498 m above sea level with passenger cabin pressurised to an altitude of 1524–2438 m.1.Cabin pressures equivalent to 2-2,500m.of altitude create a hazard of hypoxia for older travellers and place at risk those with little cardiac, cerebrovascular, respiratory reserves. Aircraft control systems maintain a pressure differential of about 9 PSI between cabin and the exterior environment. At 13,300m, the cabin is pressurised to about 2333m.and the need to fly higher to circumvent bad weather leads to a further drop in pressure. Arterial P02 at sea-level is around 9 mmHg, but at 2600m this falls to 60 mmHg in healthy young adults. Healthy passengers normally respond to pressure changes with hyperventilation and tachycardia. Those with pre-existing lung disease may not compensate adequately for the changes in atmospheric pressure in aircraft cabins .If arterial P02 levels fall to 30-40mm Hg, light exercise such as arm movements and walking may lead to dyspnoea, fatigue, light-headedness and dizziness.

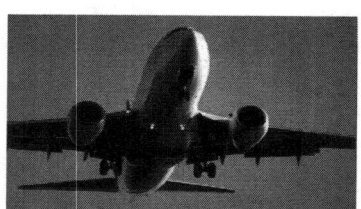

Quality of cabin air

Aviation techniques have changed over fifty years of commercial flying, but currently passengers and crew breathe air directed from the engines. When commercial flights began, passengers breathed in air supplied directly from the atmosphere using compressors. In 1962 a system was installed to draw air from the heart of the engines. "Bleed" air is drawn out of the compression section of the engine and cooled. It then enters the cabin, mixes with recirculated air passed through filters to remove bacteria and viruses. These "recirculated air" filters do not remove fumes or vapours from the engine and with a leak of hydraulic fluid, or engine oil, contamination of cabin air can theoretically occur. Most jet aircraft systems recirculate 50% of the air and top it up with fresh air. In many current aircraft the purest air often goes to the first-class section and the poorest to the rear.

Nearly all types of aircraft have been reported as affected by contaminated air, but Civil Aviation Authority (CAA) records show that British Aerospace 146, Boeing 757, Airbus A319 and the Embraer145 aeroplanes seem to be particularly susceptible. The CAA denies there is a health issue or that incidents involving fumes are not being reported. In the United States, the Federal Aviation Administration, however, noted in 2006 a serious worry about under-reporting. The Government insists there was no cover- up and that only one in 2,000 flights are affected by "fume events" and the numbers of people who reported feeling unwell as a consequence are very small. The Department of Transport is undertaking research on contaminated air in aircraft cabins.[15]

Until the last few years about 0.57 cubic metres of fresh air was provided per passenger per minute. Recently this has been about halved and more air is recirculated raising further concern about cabin contaminants, particularly carbon dioxide (CO_2) and ozone. CO_2 is produced by passengers with the quantity determined by their number and the amount of ventilation. The percentage of occupied seats therefore has a significant effect since the ventilation system is relatively limited in efficacy.

With reduction of fresh air entering the cabin, CO_2 levels have risen and may be above levels associated with comfort on some flights although within safety limits. Distribution of cabin air is not uniform, with ventilation rates in older aircraft sometimes two or three times higher in better class accommodation than in the economy section where the majority of people sit. Passenger and crew complaints of dry eyes, stuffy nose, and skin irritation, headaches, light-headedness, and confusion have been associated with cabin air quality. Chemical compounds, the result of vaporised jet oils that can mix with air have been blamed. Controlled studies on the effect of vaporised organic compounds, such as tricresyl phosphate are in progress.[16]

Episodic light headedness, headache and confusion are not uncommon occurrences in elderly people especially those on medication, which make this a difficult field to research in older travellers who may also be less tolerant of contaminated air supply.[17,18]New Boeing 787 Dreamliners coming into service use a different system to ventilate the cabin. They pump fresh air into the cabin from a source away from the engines, which ought to reduce the risk from toxic chemicals entering.

Infection in aircraft.

Atmospheric recycling within the aircraft may also theoretically increase the infectivity o f certain bacteria and viruses carried by travellers eg. influenza. This effect is made worse if closed aircraft spend long periods on the ground during delays.

Infections from serious diseases have been reported aboard commercial airlines, including influenza, [19,20,21] severe acute respiratory syndrome (SARS),[22,23] tuberculosis,[24,25] food poisoning and enteritis,[26,27,28] Air travellers travelling San Francisco to Denver during winter months showed an upper-respiratory tract infection frequency of 3–20% However travellers may acquire their viruses before rather than during the flight .[29]Congestion in airport lounges and security areas may present higher exposure to infection than time spent in an aircraft where at least some of the infective factors are filtered out. Risk of onboard transmission of infection is mainly restricted to individuals with close personal contact or, seated within two rows of an infected   passenger.[1].The risk of infection for vulnerable elderly people emphasises the wisdom of pretravel influenza and pneumococcal vaccination in susceptible elderly travellers.[18]

Air humidity and expansion of gases.

 In most aircraft fresh air is brought in from the outside, cooled and delivered to the cabin without humidification and cabin humidity can be as low as 5%. In the new Boeing 787 this will usually be 15 to 20%. Low figures may cause voice and throat problems and dehydration effects on long flights. Many older people take diuretics and may already be dehydrated compounding the effect. Overindulgence in alcohol on the journey may further add to dehydration. Air in body cavities at ground level, increases by 30% at 1830 metres altitude, to cause gastric distension and sinus problems. These changes can adversely affect the older traveller who has undergone recent surgery, gastrointestinal haemorrhage or, ear operations.

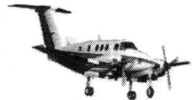

Pre-existing illness
The highest attack rates of travellers' illness are recorded in those who set off with pre-existing illness1.30 One in two individuals of 60 year olds have evidence of severe coronary arterial narrowing, although only half will have clinical signs and symptoms. Age related myocardial changes tend to present as dyspnoea rather than chest pain. A sudden breathless attack in the older traveller is likely to have a cardiac cause. Older travellers with hypertension may slip into cardiac failure if stressed. Cardiac patients frequently omit or forget to take mediation during travel and stress and strain associated with transit often results in anginal attacks and arterial occlusion. There is also a tendency for patients to avoid diuretic therapy on long journeys, which precipitates cardiac failure on prolonged flights18
In-flight deaths are relatively uncommon world-wide, but a considerable number of people of advanced years succumb to travel-induced illness in transit or immediately after air-travel. Unexpected cardiac events (myocardial infarction and ischaemia), on international flights caused 56% of in-flight fatalities. 31 One passenger in 7 million dies en route, but many are found to be seriously ill in transit airports.32 Data collation from hospitals adjacent to international airports is poor .The myocardial insufficiency in 25 people with cardiovascular problems who had collapsed in London airport had primarily occurred on the ground. Airport stress and exhaustion was considered as important a predisposing factor as in-flight hypoxia. Noise, poor communications, unexpected delay, unfamiliar melee, uncertainties of airport transit through customs, security and check-in can all dispose to confusion in older travellers 33.34
Travellers can also find themselves exposed to extremes of heat or cold at flight destinations or in unscheduled transit situations resulting from adverse weather or delay. They can also arrive at airports   situated at high altitude such as La Paz and Lhasa and be exposed to low partial pressures of environmental oxygen and suffer from hypoxia. Many older patients omit to take drugs on day of the journey   or forget to carry routine medications with them. Failure to pack regularly required drugs in hand-held luggage could precipitate cardiac and respiratory crisis in mid-air or airport.
Psychological stress
Air travel cannot be divorced from physical and psychological stressors associated with the journey to the airport, security and customs clearance, baggage handling and boarding and transfers. For many it is an anxious and even phobic experience with fears of crash, explosion and terrorist event prominent in travellers' minds. Older travellers are less capable of coping than younger people with associated transit of long walkways, physical baggage handling and the angst of delays. They become confused, fatigued and stressed, with the less fit experiencing, angina and breathlessness precipitating a cardiac event. 34,35

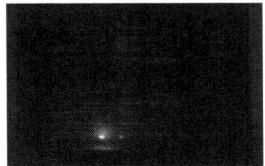
Poor communication

In-flight immobility

Many of the aged rarely leave the security of their seats while on board the aircraft. This results in accumulation of fluid in lower limbs. Gross peripheral oedema is often suffered by older passengers, during prolonged air travel. Physical constraint and immobility bring the risk of deep venous thrombosis and pulmonary embolism (PE) [36], Senescent and arthritic patients with stiff hips or fixed knees are at particular disadvantage when restricted to the narrow confines of aircraft. The need to regularly access the toilet can also put older travellers at particular risk of falls in an unstable aeroplane.

Air travel and venous thromboembolism risk

The relation between long-haul flights (more than 8 hours) and increased risk of venous remains controversial. Studies show an association between venous thromboembolism(VTE) and long-haul air travel, with risk up to four-fold,.[36][37] Risk peaks after more than 8 hours flight time[38],[39] and starts to increase when flight duration is more than 4 hours.[40] Cabin class seating has no effect on VTE incidence.[41] The greatest frequency occurs in non-aisle seating where passengers tend to move less.[42–46]

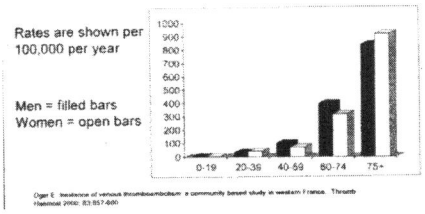

Prospective controlled cohort studies suggest a relative risk of 2•93 (95% CI1•5–5•58).[42],[44] One, a study of 9000 business travellers over 4 years, showed an absolute risk for VTE of one every 4656 flights (incidence rate ratio 3•2, 95% CI1•8–5•6).[33] Risk increases with increasing number of flights during the first 2 weeks after a flight and when other risk factors are present.

Factors increasing risk in association with air travel:-

immobility,
advancing age,
dehydration,
hypobaric hypoxia,
obesity,
malignancy,
recent surgery,

45

history of hypercoagulable states) [42,44]

One of the strongest risk factors is age with, a many times higher incidence in elderly

Additional causes of increased thrombosis in elderly people:-

Decreased mobility

Reduced muscular tone

Increased frequency of risk enhancing disease. (eg. Malignancy)

Aging tissues: Vein walls, valves and subcutaneous tissues

Immobilisation has been linked to 75% of air-travel cases of VTE; Dehydration can increase risk of venous thromboembolism due to haemoconcentration and hyperviscosity, potentially leading to hyper-coagulable states.[47]. Use of graduated compression stockings, with an ankle pressure of 17–30 mm Hg. can reduce risk during air travel. In a meta-analysis, only two of 1237 people who wore compression stockings had VTE compared with 46 of 1245 individuals who did not wear them.[48]

Anticoagulant thrombo-prophylaxis has been recommended but no formal guidelines exist. Many clinicians have recommended aspirin for individuals at moderate risk of VTE. However, evidence for benefit is scarce and risk of side effect high therefore it is not recommended alone as prophylaxis for any air traveller.[49,50] Randomised trials have shown benefit of low-molecular-weight heparin for air travellers at moderate risk of VTE and not taking routine anticoagulant drugs,[51] Routine use should be for those at high risk and be based on customised individual assessment.

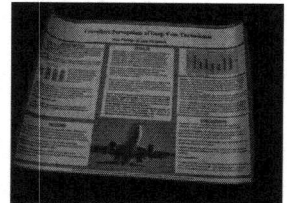

Jet lag

Air travel may prove to be an endurance test for the fit, but time zone changes and disturbance to circadian rhythm can have serious consequences for the less healthy. Time zone changes especially west to east and the crossing of three or more time zones can disturb mental alertness and cause disorientation, particularly in the old. .

Jet lag is a temporary circadian-rhythm disorder associated with long-haul flights due to desynchronisation between the body's internal clock mechanism, residing within the suprachiasmatic nucleus of the hypothalamus, and the new light–dark cycle caused by abrupt time-zonechanges.[52-4]

Symptoms are:-

- *daytime fatigue,*
- *sleep–wake disturbances,*
- *decreased appetite,*
- *constipation,*
- *reduced psychomotor coordination*
- *reduced cognitiveskills.*[52-4]

The degree and severity of jet lag is influenced by both flight direction and time zones crossed. Westward travel lengthens the day, causing a phase delay in circadian rhythm. Eastward travel shortens the day and causes a phase advance. Travellers have greater

difficulty falling asleep after eastward travel than after westward travel because of the internal clock's natural tendency to resist shortening the 24-hour day cycle
Re- synchronisation takes one day for every time zone crossed westward or 1•5 days for every time zone crossed eastward. 54.55

Limited toilet access
Elderly people have legitimate concerns about bladder function, associated with bladder and uterine prolapse and urinary frequency in the case of women and hyperprostatism and frequency in men. There can be limited toilet access in foreign airports and very limited access in aeroplanes. Queues to enter the toilet are standard on most long haul flights in economy class, which add to anxiety relating to bladder relief. Many seniors reduce fluid intake and miss out diuretic medication on the day of travel to try to reduce this problem, with resultant cardiac problems or peripheral oedema. The inadequacy of toilet access will not be addressed by airlines and seems likely to worsen if passengers are n not be addressed by airlines and seems likely to worsen if passengers are not allowed to access toilets in the hour before landing, which has happened recently in aircraft landing in the USA. Prostatic obstruction and urinary retention related to travel is not uncommon and is a worry for many older male travellers. Health professionals should be aware of these concerns and potential problems, offer counselling and encourage routine uptake of diuretics during travel.

Advice for potential Elderly air travellers.
VTE Avoidance
Low risk
Flight time less than 8 h or distance less than 5000 km and fit ,slim passengers
Avoid constrictive clothing
avoid dehydration;
move about cabin when possible
do calf-stretching exercises
Moderate risk
Flight time more than 8 h or distance more than 5000 km
Where obesity, large varicose veins, hormone-replacement therapy, tobacco use relative immobility are considerations
Low-risk measures plus
 properly fitted below-knee compression stockings providing 15–30 mm Hg of pressure at the ankle;
aisle seating
High risk
Flight time more than 8 h or distance more than 5000 km
With history of previous venous thromboembolism; hypercoagulable state (egfactor V Leiden); major surgery 6 weeks before air travel (including hip or knee arthroplasty);known malignancy
Low and Moderate-risk measures and:
low-molecular-weight heparin injected before departure in people not on warfarin
Contraindications to commercial air travel
Total contraindications to flying on scheduled services are few and delay in departure date may allow acceptance of those temporary unfit. People must refrain from high flying, however, if they suffer from a disease adversely affected by hypoxia or pressure changes

produced by altitude. Those with little cardiac, cerebrovascular and respiratory reserves can meet with problems. In general, dyspnoea at rest is a contraindication to prolonged air travel. Patients with severe anaemia and within two weeks of myocardial infarction occurrence, cerebrovascular accident, or in cardiac failure should not indulge in travel. Alternative routing or trip or even cancellation may be advisable.

Medical fitness for air travel

Airlines have the right to refuse passengers who are unfit to fly for medical reasons.[6,56] Passengers should be able to walk a distance of 50 m and climb one flight of stairs without angina or severe dyspnoea.[6]

Conditions which are excluded for immediate travel by airlines:-

- Cardiac conditions

Unstable angina

Myocardial infarction occurring 7–10 days before air travel

Uncontrolled dysrhythmia

Coronary artery bypass graft operation 10–14 days before air travel

Decompensated heart failure

- Respiratory conditions

Baseline sea-level $PaO_2 < 67–70$ mm Hg without supplemental oxygen

Exacerbation of moderate obstructive/restrictive lung-disease

Contagious pulmonary infections

Large pleural effusion

Pneumothorax 3 weeks before air travel

- Neurological disorders

• Stroke within 5–10 days of travel

• Uncontrolled seizures or 24–hours after grand-mal seizure

- Surgical interventions

A gastrointestinal, thoracic, ear, nose, and throat, and neurological surgical procedure 10–14 days before air travel

laparoscopic surgery 5 days before air travel

On board Medical Assistance

In 1 in 50 international flights medical help is requested in three out of four in-flight emergencies, there is a physician on board when it occurs.[1] Commercial aircraft carry 1-4 medical kits and at least one enhanced emergency medical kit, required by aviation regulation Most commercial flights also carry an automated external defibrillator. Some commercial air carriers use on-ground tele-medical assistance to medically assess passengers who seem unfit for travel at boarding. This service can provide medical advice during in-flight medical events service can provide medical advice during in-flight medical events providing 24-hour ground-to-air medical support and advising the flight deck on best diversion location and emergency personnel availability. Elderly passengers should be made aware that illness on an aircraft is an experience best avoided. Attending doctors may have limited or unpractised emergency skills and are limited by resources and space in providing an optimum therapeutic response

Pre-flight assessment

Many airlines have that if a passenger is fit enough to walk up steps into the aircraft, he or she is fit to fly. Modern airport design means that passengers seldom need to climb steps, but should however be able to walk 50 metres on the flat without breathlessness. In passengers who can just manage this feat there may still be doubt about their fitness to travel. More scientific assessment may require referral to a respiratory unit. If simple spirometry and blood gases are known and the patient has chronic obstructive airways disease (COAD), an idea of oxygenation at altitude can be obtained from a hypoxia challenge test.

The hypoxia challenge test involves the patient breathing 15% oxygen in nitrogen and measuring saturation. This gas mixture simulates oxygen available in the aircraft cabin at maximum cruising altitude. If saturation falls below 85% during test then in-flight oxygen will be required. This test also allows assessment of symptoms that may arise at a lesser degree of hypoxaemia. Eg the patient with coronary artery disease who gets angina during the hypoxic challenge even though the fall in saturation on its own would not be regarded as severe enough to require oxygen. This patient too would require continuous in-flight oxygen to prevent angina during flight.[57]

Oxygen supplementation is recommended for passengers with either a resting oxygen saturation of 92% or lower (PaO_2=67 mm Hg) or if the expected in-fl ight PaO_2 is less than 50–55 mm Hg.[9] The American Aerospace Medical Association recommends in-flight oxygen for individuals with a sea-level PaO_2 of 70 mm Hg or lower, or an expected in-flight PaO_2 of 55 mm Hg or lower.[10] Guidelines from the British Thoracic Society (BTS)[13] suggest hypoxic-challenge testing in individuals with resting oxygen saturations of 92–95% at sea level who have additional risk factors, such as hypercapnia or abnormal spirometry.

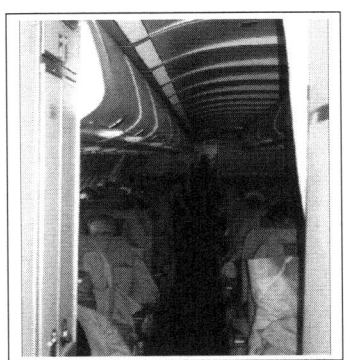

Practical recommendations for all older travellers
- Carry routine medications in hand luggage
- Travel with spare medications
- Take medications as normal unless advised otherwise by travel health counsellor
- Carry a list of routine medications for information of emergency personnel
- Maintain good hydration,
- Reduce alcohol and caffeine consumption en route
- Walk in the cabin when possible and stroll about departure lounges.
- Periodically exercise calf-muscles when sitting en route

- Use compression stockings if at higher risk of VTE or prone to immobility and put them on when recumbent before leaving home.
- If moderately breathless at rest, seek pre travel health assessment from a doctor
- A passenger needing supplementary oxygen, requires physician documentation stating fitness to travel at 2438 m altitude
- Passengers who have had surgery or a pneumothorax within 2 weeks are at risk of retained pockets of air expanding and causing problems and should seek pretravel medical advice.
- Passengers with colostomies are advised to use a large bag and to carry a spare!
- Advise the airline by using the Medif form of any potential medical or mobility problems before travel.
- Utilise wheelchairs, moving footways and invalid transport where at all possible in airports.
- Consider business class travel if affordable for enhanced comfort on aeroplanes and in lounges.

Jet lag precautions

Pre-flight sleep preparation:-
Westbound:
Go to sleep 1 hour later than usual
Rise 1 hour later than usual 3 days before travelling•
Eastbound:
Go to sleep 1 hour earlier than usual
be awake 1 hour earlier than usual 3 days before travelling
Exogenous melatonin is recommended.
Taken in the evening, melatonin phase advances the circadian clock,
early morning administration ,phase delays the circadian rhythm.
Cochrane meta-analysis concluded that taking 0•5–5 mg of melatonin at the desired destination bedtime is effective for reducing or preventing jet lag.
Use of *bright-light exposure* to adjust circadian rhythm is still being researched.
Recommended especially if crossing five or more time zones, travelling eastwardly, or with a history of jet-lag symptoms. Caution is required in people with epilepsy or on warfarin
Benzodiazepines
Some reported efficacy in sleep quality (eg, temazepam) and other circadian-rhythm or sleep parameters, although sleeping medication increase the likelihood of immobility and may therefore increase the risk of VTE development.

References

1 Silverman D, Gendreau M .Medical issues associated with commercial flights www.thelancet.com Published online February 19, 2009 DOI:10.1016/S0140-6736(09)60209-9
2 British Airports Authority. Audit and development Annual report 2007
3 Cummings R. Chapman P. 1988 In-flight deaths during commercial air travel J. Amer. Med. Assoc. 259,13,1983-88
4 Woods D 1991 Medical hazards of flying Med. Monitor. 5.4
5 Cocks R, Liew M. Commercial aviation in-flight emergencies and the physician. Emerg Med Australas 2007; 19: 1–8.
6 Tonks A. Cabin fever. BMJ 2008; 336: 584–86
7 Gendreau MA, DeJohn C. Responding to medical events during commercial airline flights. N Engl J Med 2002; 346: 1067–73.
8 DeJohn CA, Wolbrink AM, Veronneau SJ, Larcher JG, Smith DW,Garrett JS. An evaluation of in-flight medical care in the U.S. Aviat Space Environ Med 2002; 73: 580–86.
9 Cabin cruising altitudes for regular transport aircraft.Aviat Space Environ Med 2008; 79: 433–39.
10 Toff WD, Jones CI, Ford I, et al. Eff ect of hypobaric hypoxia,simulating conditions during long-haul air travel, on coagulation, fibrinolysis, platelet function, and endothelial activation. JAMA2006; 295: 2251–61.

11 Seccombe LM, Peters MJ. Oxygen supplementation for chronic obstructive pulmonary disease patients during air travel.Curr Opin Pulm Med 2006; 12: 140–44.

12 Burnett JC. Long- and short-haul travel by air: issues for people with diabetes on insulin J.Trav. Med.2006.13.255-60

13 Managing passengers with respiratory disease planning air travel: British Thoracic Society recommendations. Thorax 2002; 57: 289–304.

14 Cabin cruising altitudes for regular transport aircraft.Aviat Space Environ Med 2008; 79: 433–39.

15 Air Travel and Health Report. House of Lords Select cttee. on Sc. and tech.201 HMSO

16 Humphreys S, Deyermond R, Bali I, Stevenson M, Fee JP. The effect of high altitude commercial air travel on oxygen saturation. Anaesthesia 2005; 60: 458–60.

17 McIntosh I Travel and Health in the elderly .1992 Quay Books Publishing. Lancaster

18 McIntosh I The vulnerable, older traveller 2009 CME Geriatric Med.11(3)118-22

19 Evans A, Finkelstein S, Singh J, Thibeault C. Pandemic influenza:a note on international planning to reduce the risk from air transport. Aviat Space Environ Med 2006; 77: 974–76.

20 Moser MR, Bender TR, Margolis HS, Noble GR, Kendal AP,Ritter DG. An outbreak of infl uenza aboard a commercial airliner. Am J Epidemiol 1979; 110: 1–6.

21 Marsden AG. Outbreak of influenza-like illness related to air travel. Med J Aust 2003; 179: 172–73. 189 (suppl 1): S81–85.

22 Olsen SJ, Chang HL, Cheung TY, et al. Transmission of the severe acute respiratory syndrome on aircraft. N Engl J Med 2003; 349: 2416–22.

23 Wilder-Smith A, Leong HN. A case of in-flight transmission of severe acute respiratory syndrome (SARS): SARS serology positive. J Travel Med 2004; 11: 130.

24 McFarland JW, Hickman C, Osterholm M, MacDonald KL.Exposure to Mycobacterium tuberculosis during air travel. Lancet 1993; 342: 112–13.

25 Exposure of passengers and flght crew to Mycobacterium tuberculosis on commercial aircraft, 1992–1995.MMWR Morb Mortal Wkly Rep 1995; 44: 137–40.

26Tauxe RV, Tormey MP, Mascola L, Hargrett-Bean NT, Blake PA.Salmonellosis outbreak on transatlantic fl ights; foodborne illness on aircraft: 1947–1984. Am J Epidemiol 1987; 125: 150–57.

27 McMullan R, Edwards PJ, Kelly MJ, Millar BC, Rooney PJ,Moore JE. Food-poisoning and commercial air travel.Travel Med Infect Dis 2007; 5: 276–86.

28 Widdowson MA, Glass R, Monroe S, et al. Probable transmission ofnorovirus on an airplane. JAMA 2005; 293: 1859–60.

29 Zitter JN, Mazonson PD, Miller DP, Hulley SB, Balmes JR. Aircraft cabin air recirculation and symptoms of the common cold. JAMA2002; 288: 483–86.

30 McIntosh I Travel Induced illness Scot. Med. 1991.11. 14-15

31 Agostoni P, Cattadori G, Guazzi M, et al. Effects of simulated altitude-induced hypoxia on exercise capacity in patients with chronic heart failure. Am J Med 2000; 109: 450–55.

32 Erdmann J, Sun KT, Masar P, Niederhauser H. Eff ects of exposureto altitude on men with coronary artery disease and impaired leftventricular function. Am J Cardiol 1998; 81: 266–70.

33 McIntosh I 1990 The stress of modern travel Trav Med Internat.118 18-24

34 McIntosh I Power K. et al. Prevalence and intensity of travel related stressors J Trav Med. 1996 3(2)96-102

35 McIntosh I Power K Anxiety and Health problems related to air travel . J Trav Med.1998 12. 40-3

36 Becker NG, SalIM A, Kelman CW. Air travel and the risk of deep vein thrombosis. Aust NZ J Public Health 2006; 30: 5–9.

37 Schwarz T, Siegert G, Oettler W, et al. Venous thrombosis after long-haul fl ights. Arch Intern Med 2003; 163: 2759–64.

38 Hughes R, Heuser T, Hill S, et al. Recent air travel and venous thromboembolisim (NZATT) study. Lancet 2003; 362: 2039–44.

40 Cannegieter SC, Doggen CJ, van Houwelingen HC, Rosendaal FR.Travel-related venous thrombosis: results from a large population-based case control study (MEGA study). PLoS Med 2006;

41 Jacobson BF, Munster M, Smith A, et al. The BEST study–a prospective study to compare business class versus economy class air travel as a cause of thrombosis. S Afr Med J 2003; 93: 522–28.

42 Philbrick JT, Shumate R, Siadaty MS, Becker DM. Air travel andvenous thromboembolism: a systematic review. J Gen Intern Med 2007; 22: 107–14.

43 Trujillo-Santos AJ, Jimenez-Puente A, Perea-Milla E. Association between long travel and venous thromboembolic disease: a systematic review and meta-analysis of case-control studies. Ann Hematol 2008; 87: 79–86.

44 Aryal KR, Al-Khaff af H. Venous thromboembolic complications following air travel: what's the quantitative risk? A literature review. Eur J Vasc Endovasc Surg 2006; 31: 187–99.

45 Kuipers S, Schreijer AJ, Cannegieter SC, Buller HR, Rosendaal FR,Middeldorp S. Travel and venous thrombosis: a systematic review.

46Tasker A, Akinola O, Cohen AT. Review of venous thromboembolism associated with air travel. Travel Med Infect Dis 2004; 2: 75–79.

47 Bendz B, Rostrup M, Sevre K, Andersen TO, Sandset PM.Association between acute hypobaric hypoxia and activation of coagulation in human beings. Lancet 2000; 356: 1657–58.

48 Hsieh HF, Lee FP. Graduated compression stockings as prophylaxisfor flight-related venous thrombosis: systematic literature review.J Adv Nurs 2005; 51: 83–98.

49 Geerts WH, Bergqvist D, Pineo GF, et al. Prevention of venous thromboembolism: American College of Chest Physicians Evidence-Based Clinical Practice Guidelines (8th edn). Chest 2008; 133 (suppl): 381S–453S.

50 Watson HG, Chee YL. Aspirin and other antiplatelet drugs in the prevention of venous thromboembolism. Blood Rev 2008; 22: 107–16.

51 Chee YL, Watson HG. Air travel and thrombosis. Br J Haematol2005; 130: 671–80

52 Sadun AA, Schaechter JD, Smith LE. A retinohypothalamic pathwayin man: light mediation of circadian rhythms. Brain Res 1984; 302: 371–77.

53 Saper CB, Lu J, Chou TC, Gooley J. The hypothalamic integrator for circadian rhythms. Trends Neurosci 2005; 28: 152–57.

54 Dubocovich ML. Melatonin receptors: role on sleep and circadian rhythm regulation. Sleep Med 2007; 8 (suppl 3): 34–42.

55 Revell VL, Eastman CI. How to trick mother nature into letting you fly around or stay up all night. J Biol Rhythms 2005; 20: 353–65.

55 Sack RL, Auckley D, Auger RR, et al. Circadian rhythm sleep disorders: part I, basic principles, shift work and jet lag disorders. An American Academy of Sleep Medicine review. Sleep 2007; 30: 1460–83.

56 Jorge A, Pombal R, Peixoto H, Lima M. Preflight medical clearance of ill and incapacitated passengers: 3-year retrospective study of experience with a European airline. J Travel Med 2005; 12: 306–11.

57 Dine CJ, Kreider ME. Hypoxia altitude simulation test. Chest 2008;133: 1002–05.

Iain B.McIntosh

Chapter 5

Land and Sea Travel and Associated Illness

Sea Travel

In the last decade there has been a huge increase in sea and river cruising. Fly-cruising has become very popular, with passengers flying from Britain to board vessels berthed in ports across the globe. Elderly passengers in particular have embraced sea cruising, attracted by its luxury, protected environment, access to far distant destinations and 24 hour per day, on board medical attention. Cruise ships travel regularly to the Arctic, Antarctica across the Pacific and Atlantic oceans and up the world's great rivers.

They disembark passengers in exotic ports; remote islands unexplored gulfs, congested conurbations and disease-ridden destinations. Their human cargo pours into major cities with excellent medical facilities and into undeveloped areas of the Third World, with poor health resources and scant emergency aid for foreign visitors. The voyager can be exposed to, malaria, exotic disease, infected water and food and trauma.

Many of these passengers are elderly people with ships carrying a large number of senior citizens, many in imperfect health. They travel with pre-existing illness, taking several medications, with scant knowledge of health risk, resources and facilities, at ports visited en route. They are unaware of limited facilities available to on-board medical staff and the inadequacies of health care and evacuation, they might meet in emergency.

The majority indulge in maritime adventure and return home in good health, but health insurance claims from older travellers continue to rise. Travel health professionals need to be aware of the risks to which elderly travellers are exposed, precautions they should take before and during travel and prophylaxis and vaccination to reduce health risk.

Ever-bigger ships are being launched. Some can accommodate 5,000 passengers and they venture to more adventurous and exotic locations. World-wide over 12 million people cruise the high seas annually visiting 2000 ports. One million Britons cruised in 2005. [1]
Mediterranean and Caribbean Seas are most popular destinations with average cruise 7-14 days. World cruises last months and many elderly people stay aboard for 6 weeks or more. Overall health and safety record is good, but ships are inherently unstable and operate in regions where there is hazard to health. They are potential transmission sources and reservoirs for infection. Infection and injury befall passengers, especially the frail and elderly. [2,3]

Older Passengers

Elderly people are the second largest group to long haul destinations.[4] The type of itinerary affects passenger risk, with deep sea, ocean, large river e.g. Amazon/Orinoco, polar, adventure cruising, presenting different health hazards. A cruise ship is a global community, a closed, air-conditioned environment with potential for disease exposure. Rapid movement between ports with varying sanitation standards and disease exposure can introduce communicable disease, with spread of infection in a crowded vessel. Shipboard living may become a problem for old passengers, if they have exacerbation of chronic illness or an acute event.[5] One third of passengers are over 60 years age and in some ships three quarters are over 65 yrs. The majority are middle aged and above and many have preexisting medical disorders.[2]

Passenger morbidity
Warm water cruising

Incidence of disease and medical intervention depends upon conditions of sea, climate, ship size, passenger age and sex. [6.7.8]. Many passengers are injured ashore. Data considered commercially sensitive, is limited and often relates to single ships, or cruises. On average, on a one week cruise to the Caribbean, medical staff will be consulted by up to-55 passengers, with 80-90% infirmary visits for non-urgent conditions.10-15% will be urgent,5-10% for serious illness or injury requiring on board hospitalisation or evacuation. 1% of ship patients require emergency transfer to shore based hospital. [9.3] One in every 250 passengers experiences a serious illness that requires in patient care. [10]

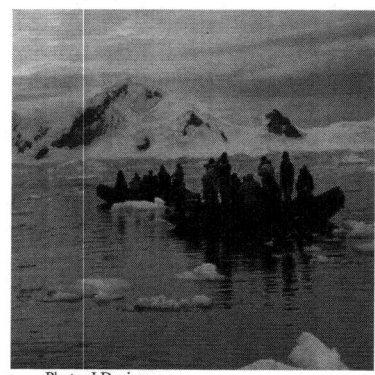

Photo. J.Davies

Cold water cruises

There were 9,322 tourists in1996 to the Antarctic .In years 1998-2000, four ships carried 3,637 passengers on Antarctic cruises of 15 days. The majority of passengers were 64-74 years old. Older passengers did not consult the doctor more frequently, but had more serious illnesses and injuries than younger travellers. Consultation rate was 33.1 consultations per 1000 passenger days in Antarctic, as opposed to 4.6 warm water cruises.50.5% of passengers consulted the doctor on polar cruises compared to 3.6% on warm water ones.[12]

The spectrum of disease is similar in cruise ships to Arctic and Antarctica, with significant increase in sea sickness in the Antarctic. The proportion of passengers consulting the doctor was similar for polar regions, but much less in warm water cruising.[13] Consultation rate was 33.1 consultations per 1000 passenger days in Antarctica as opposed to 4.6 for warm water cruise.50.5% of passengers consulted the doctor on polar cruises compared to 3.6% on warm water ones.[12] Over 60 % consultations in Antarctic were for seasickness Respiratory illness was second most common presentation in Arctic [13.4] and Antarctic-5%- and most common in warm waters. [14.15] There was no significant additional medical risk for passengers cruising polar waters. Cold injury (1%) was uncommon in people cruising in Antarctica. Patients with illness and injury may have to remain on board for some time in heavy seas in polar waters.[16]

Passenger morbidity [14.17]

Condition	%
Respiratory	26-29
Injury related-	12-18
Gastro-intestinal	12-16
Cardiovascular	3-7
Skin	3-13

In 5215 passenger presentations to ship doctors over 20 cruises the most common presentations were respiratory (18%), circulatory (13%) injury (12%). One in three had seasickness. Seasickness, respiratory problems and injuries accounted for 72%. [20]Contusions, lacerations and burns were common injuries with, lower limbs affected in passengers. Contusions were most frequent representing 1/3 of all injuries. In a further study most frequent illnesses were respiratory, seasickness and gastro-intestinal disease.[21.22] Medical intervention was requested for virus infection, hypertension, sea-sickness, injuries, and chronic disease in elderly passengers.[23] On 35 cruises, 35 passengers were hospitalised, 4 with myocardial infarction, 2 with peptic ulcer perforations. [24]

Deaths aboard ship

In a 6-year study of passenger mortality on two ships (complement 88 passengers), 25 died, with an average of one death per 6 months per ship. More men than women died (P>0.05).Nine died after up to 52 hours of intensive on board care. Five had cardiac problems,. Findings were similar on four larger ships studied over a year.7147 passengers attended the ship's clinic in 1,537,298 passenger days with 2.6 versus 3.6 mortalities per thousand passengers per year.18% presenting had injuries, with precipitating event a slip, fall or trip. Older women were largest group to be hospitalised. 69.3% for medical conditions. Most common diagnosis was respiratory infection [21] 11% had serious or life threatening event. The spectrum of conditions was similar to hospital emergency departments. With 12% related to injury, 88% to medical problems and 3% emergency intervention.[22]

Elderly Passengers

Three cruise lines reported that 1 in 5000 passengers suffers a serious medical crisis requiring evacuation. A ship physician caring for 1000 passengers may expect potentially serious illness or injury and have to disembark people once a week.[12] People older than 64 years accounted for 51% of clinic attendees. [23]Similar results were obtained on a 103-day cruise with 3033 passengers and 693consultations. Average age was over 60 years. Passengers accounted for 59% doctor consultations, 27% of accidents to passengers occurred ashore.7 passengers were referred to shore specialists and 7 were hospitalised on land. One died aboard.

In case comparison analysis of factors associated with injuries aboard ships resulting in hospitalisations of residents and non-residents in Alaska (1991-2000) showed non-resident females, 65+ years old, were aboard cruise ships when injured. They were more likely to suffer fractures and serious injury and experience post injury disability.[24]

Small boat and rigid inflatable dinghy transfers add risk for elderly cruise passengers with ship to shore transfers from large ships to small boats inherently dangerous in cold, rough seas.Shore excursions require stamina, challenge the old. They may last 12 –13 hours and take passengers to remote spots and expose them to infection, trauma, fatigue, immobility in coaches and morbidity, especially if people are travelling with pre-existing illness. [21.25.26] Ocean cruising may be inappropriate for very elderly, frail, handicapped and mentally unprepared passengers. [27.28] Many ships now have designated cabins for the handicapped, but the inherently unstable, hazardous environment will pose special risk for these people who would be particular challenged in a disaster situation.

Risks to Health in Cruise travel
Infection
Trauma
UVL exposure
Motion sickness
Air transit problems

Cruise infections
Infection can occur :-
en route to embarkation.
on board. Bacteria and viruses introduced by crew, passengers and ship systems result in
- Influenza and para influenzal illness
- diarrhoea,
- Legionnaires disease,
- Rubella, all of which can spread rapidly

on, shore excursions which expose passengers to :-
- Local and exotic infection
- Malaria
- Dengue fever
- Food and water borne infection
- Insect borne disease
- Infection from bites

on return home.
Risk of exposure to infectious disease is difficult to quantify because of the broad spectrum of cruise ships and itineraries and limited data on infectious diseases occurring on ships.[29] Cruise lines are loath to publicise data. Surveillance systems have identified cases of food poisoning:-
Norwalk virus, Legionella Influenza A and B infections, chicken pox and measles. [12]
Legionella pneumonophilia can cause severe pneumonia and even death in the frail and elderly. Legionella species enter ship potable systems. The organism needs poor chlorination or temperature control to multiply. [30]In a Case control study, among 215 passengers to the North Cape, 45 were affected and one died. The source was prolonged exposure to in the spa pool. [31]Outbreaks have been associated with ship spas, fountains and showers which generate aerosols necessary for spread of disease.[12] Inhalation of aerosols contaminated with Legionella bacteria often occurs in the whirlpool spa.[32] A prevalence study on 9 cruise ships and ferries revealed 42% of water supplies were contaminated by Legionella species. Legionella is a ubiquitous organism that can survive in ship board freshwater systems.[33] In specimens from showers and washbasins L. pneumonophilia was isolated in 95.5% samples.
Influenza A and B. Influenzal outbreaks have occurred on cruise ships worldwide. Although cruise ships were not actual source they became a reservoir of infection. There is recorded increased morbidity on cruise ships.There have been prolonged outbreaks of both influenza A and B with fatalities in Caribbean ,Pacific Alaska and Mediterranean.[34,35,36]
Gastro-intestinal illness (AGE) is common, comprising 5-10% of sick bay visits. Some is due to ingestion of water and food partaken off the ship. Half the cases are due to Norwalk virus the rest enterotoxic E. Coli(ETEC), salmonella, shigella, staphylococcus aureus and campylobacter [37,38] Norovirus infection is difficult to eradiate in cruise ships where rapid

transmission can occur between passengers, It is not usually serious ,although elderly people can become dehydrated and require fluid replacement. Symptoms arise 24-48 hours after exposure and illness lasts 1-4 days. It is transmitted through contact with infected persons, poor hygiene, or the handling of contaminated objects. Raw or undercooked shellfish and chilled foods, including salads and sandwiches, can become a source of infection.

In 2002- there was a sharp increase in norovirus associated illness on ships and land.[39] In 14 laboratory confirmed outbreaks on ships, [12](86%) were attributed to calciviruses with continuation on successive cruises, multiple methods of transmission and high attack rates (58%) CDC Atlanta recorded 21 outbreaks of acute gastroenteritis (AGE) on 17 ships, 9 associated with noroviruses, 3 to bacterial agents and 9 of unknown aetiology

In 2003-600 passengers were infected on two ships. 2% passengers and 7% crew had AGE illness. Another vessel with 2250 passengers was also affected with same virus. 200 passengers were infected and confined to cabins for 4 days. 3 other ships and the worlds largest liner –were affected on Caribbean cruises.

Ship board out breaks of Norwalk infection have been caused by ice, shrimps, fresh fruit . Intensive ship cleaning does not always eradicate the infection.(12)In cruises of 3 – 15 days there are 1.4 outbreaks of diarrhoeal disease per 1000 cruises or 2.3 outbreaks per 10 million passenger days, or 6 outbreak related illnesses per 100,000 passenger days. Between 1986-93, 5278 passengers were affected. Most common source was undercooked scallops, eggs and food taken on shore excursions. –thorough cooking of sea foods and use of pasteurised eggs would have reduced the infection by half.[40] Enterotoxic E. Coli infection has been sourced to ingested and consumption of fresh cut fruit and water bunkering in transit ports.[41]

In 2005 a report revealed poor hygiene practices and health hazards on random checks on 14 British cruise ships docking in British ports . There has been a call for Britain to follow the USA to publish cruise ship hygiene reports by ports inspectors.[42]

Accidents and Injuries

An agency offering ship physician assistance reported on 1700 cases on 500 different ships. 65% were due to illness and 33% injury, which included musculoskeletal (21%) skin trauma (15%), 13% were eventually repatriated..

• Most frequent cause of ship accidents are stairways, gangways, decks ,slippery surfaces
• Unfamiliar environment causes many accidents, especially in the elderly with poor balance disturbed gait and locomotion difficulties.
• Sprains and contusions are most frequently reported injuries.
• Common reported accidents are falls/cuts/grazes.
• 66% of all accidents are preventable

Temperatures below +20 degrees C met in polar cruising, increase unsafe behaviour. Cold causes clumsiness and decreases muscle strength. [12]

Inhalation injuries constitute the main risk with on board fire. Fast airstreams develop in corridors and air ducts. Lack of oxygen below decks occurs early in the fire and smoke and fumes contain chemical elements of incomplete burning. Survival and injury depend upon the location of the ship, proximity of other rescue ships and sea state. People have a better chance of survival on a burnt out ship than in a lifeboat.

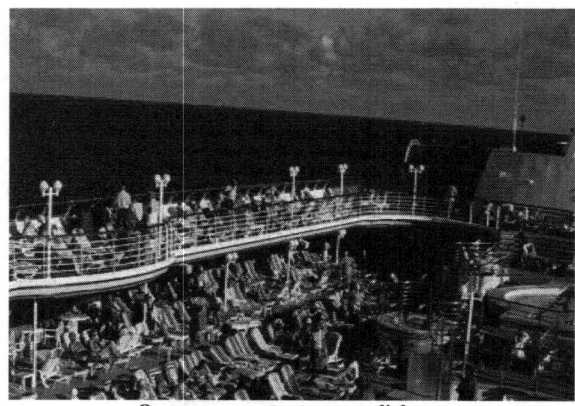
Over-exposure to strong sunlight

Ultraviolet light over exposure
Many passengers over expose themselves to strong sunlight on cruises with adverse solar effects compounded by reflection from the sea. Others, especially the old, fall asleep in the sun and are badly burnt. Solar radiation over Antarctica is four times greater than where earth is protected by atmospheric ozone. [11]

Sea sickness
100% of passengers were affected in rough conditions in the Southern Ocean [14] and motion sickness can affect many people, even on ships with stabilisers [3] severe vomiting results in dehydration and interference with routine medication .It is perhaps less likely to affect passengers with mid-ship, mid-deck in board cabins. Favoured drugs are cinnarizine ,scopolamine and promethazine.[20,21] Only 1/3 of sea- sick passengers ask for medical help [19,43] Anti sea-sickness medication has a 30% positive placebo [44]

On-board medical facilities.
Cruise lines strive to maintain a healthy, safe on-board environment. Most large ships have excellent medical facilities, but cannot equate with on shore hospitals. There are no international standards of care for cruise ships. In 1990 the American College of Emergency Physicians (ACEP) Cruise ship and Maritime Medicine section was founded to :-Act as a resource for cruise industry physicians and departments and develop guidelines,(GLs). Many ships have medical staffing and facilities in accordance with ACEP, GLs but they do not provide emergency surgery, blood transfusion, extensive laboratory or radiological services. The ship's physician position is determined by "custom", not maritime law and many are employed as independent contractors. Except for ships registered in Norway and England there are no mandatory international maritime requirements for cruise lines to carry a licensed physician, or have hospital facilities aboard. but ships carrying over 50 passengers generally have both. Quality of facilities, medical practice and physician varies depending upon itinerary, ships complement and construction
North Americans staff about 10% of cruise ship medical rooms, Staff manage severe blood loss with fluid replacement using IV colloids and crystalloids as they do not carry blood products.[14]Most shipboard physicians are not certified in trauma treatment or medical evacuation. There is no internationally agreed standard relating to certification. Most ship

doctors are general practitioners on short-term contracts. This can lead to poor continuity and variable standards. The ACEP health care GLs may not be followed by smaller ships, or those run by independent companies where there may be limited medical facilities on board, sometimes located in the doctor's cabin. The ratio of medical staff to passengers varies greatly from ship to ship with one of 88 passengers having a doctor and a nurse and the large Carnival line ships of 3000 passengers having also only one doctor eg." QE2" with 2921 passengers has a doctor, surgeon and 6 nurses while the "Sensation" with 3541 passengers has one doctor and 2 nurses.

Shipboard medical centres are not hospitals and should be considered first aid stations for temporary stabilisation until shore side facilities are reached, a fact rarely appreciated by passengers The cruise line is liable for physician's negligence in treatment of crew but not in treatment of passengers, providing it endeavoured to hire a competent doctor.

Ship Pharmacy Medications
Medications stocked on board vary markedly from ship to ship and record systems for availability and expiry can be poor with an ever-changing professional resource.. ACEP, Gls encourage standardised equipment, supplies and medications, but cruise lines do not have to comply. Ships often have no oxygen –saturation monitor to determine blood oxygen levels although standard in most land based emergency departments. Gls. for handling emergencies vary from ship to ship with many having elaborate well-rehearsed emergency response systems and others ad hoc arrangements Disaster drills though realistic can be counterproductive, with the launching of lifeboats on compulsory passenger drills causing more harm than occurs in real disasters.

Disabled passengers
A cruise ship is not a safe environment for some travellers but there are few embarkation restrictions. Unqualified or poorly trained medical staff and/ inadequate medical equipment are serious risk factors for ill or injured passengers. (14)Newer ships are more accessible for people with disabilities. At present only 4 cruise ships give direct ramp access to lifeboats. Specially trained crew members have to be trained to assist wheelchair passengers - 2 per 8 hour shift according to latest safety and evacuation regulations

Fly cruising
Many passengers now undertake long and medium haul air travel en route to the ship and are posed to health risks associated with long air journeys. The precautions for long haul flights to avoid deep vein thrombosis apply. See Chapter 4.)

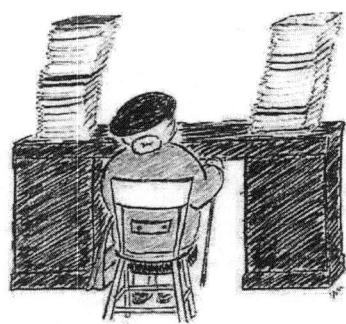

Pretravel Risk assessment. It is essential that pre travel risk assessment is undertaken and pre-travel advice given to the elderly and chronically ill. Risks may be reduced by ensuring passengers understand potential hazards, especially during rough seas.
If a person is very unfit, with serious medical problems and easily confused a cruising holiday may not be in their best interest. [45]
People in poor health or with a history of recurrent serious and chronic illness should pick voyages with short distances between ports with good facilities.
Effective emergency plans; aggressive treatment of serious medical conditions and proactive evacuation policy will keep the number of deaths at sea low. [46]
Targeted safety promotion regarding potential injury is required for elderly people, especially females. [43]

Travellers on board cruise ships should be prepared for the possibility of illness and injury and realise that even minor injury may require evacuation to shore facilities. They should appreciate the limitation of medical facilities and providers on board ship and that continuing care will depend on the nearest port with variable shore. [34]
Check List for passengers
Passengers should:-
*   buy adequate and comprehensive travel health insurance
*   enquire about the size of ship, distance between ports, quality of medical staff and facilities.
*   choose a cruise with close proximity of ports and good evacuation possibilities if likely to require emergency care.
*   be aware that ship medical rooms should be considered first aid stations for temporary stabilisation until shore side facilities are reached,
*   remember quality of continuing medical care is dependent upon that available at first port of call
*   carry anti-emetic medication ,a list of medications and medical history, adequate routine medications, antidiarrhoeal and antimetic preparations, sun block
*   have pre travel influenza and pneumococcal vaccine prophylaxis
*   Immunity compromised passengers e.g.. splenectomised, IV infected, or taking steroids or immuno suppressive therapy should be aware of infection risk.
*   Acquire a note from family doctor recording medical history and medications
*   Carry adequate supplies of medications on the person en route and on excursions.

- If subject to motion sickness passengers should seek mid-ship, mid-deck inner cabins and adopt supine position parallel to ship axis of major motion, to minimises effects of motion on vestibular apparatus, in rough seas.
- Be aware of risk of enteritis infection from salads, shell food on board
- Take advantage of alcohol based aerosol antibacterial hand washes provided for embarking passengers and those arriving for meals.
- Be chary of on shore infected water and food
- Remember that on fly cruises the precautions for safe air travel also apply

Recommended Medications
Favoured drugs for motion sickness are cinnarizine, scopolamine and promethazine.[43,44]
Influenzal immunisation
Pneumococcal immunisation
Antimalarials where appropriate

Land Travel
Many ships berth in a different port every day and disgorge passengers for a day of exploration on land. They voyage to many destinations in undeveloped parts of the world where transport and roads can be rudimentary and road traffic accidents common. Many day trippers take the opportunity to tour the local town and hinterland by coach, on local buses or hire cars. They take to this transport without thought regarding the health risk to which they may be exposed.[45]
On vacation and relaxed they forget simple precautions for road safety they practice at home. They enter vehicles which are not roadworthy and walk highways without regard for personal safety. They hire, beach vehicles, safari cars, motor bikes and scooters and ride them without helmets or seat belts. They often transit over poorly constructed roads and maintained roads with low safety margins, in mountainous and jungle terrain. They jaywalk and traverse poorly maintained pavements and many do so having imbibed freely on local alcoholic spirit.
Older passengers compound potential safety risk with systemic failings interfering with balance, gait and agility and disability interfering with mobility. Forgetting their years they unwisely enter rickshaws and tuk tuks to be driven by young drivers inured to accident risk, unaware that road traffic accident is likely possibility in foreign travel.[46,47]
Statistics show that the chances of being involved in a car accident however in mainland Europe doubles, and it almost triples in Greece and Portugal and double and treble for undeveloped countries of Asia and the Caribbean.[48]Accidents cause 20% of all deaths among overseas travellers – the second most common cause after heart disease (68%)
Many holiday accident claims occur before holiday makers even make their destinations as the UK national estimate for accidents while travelling and touring was 480,664 in 2008
Older drivers are more likely to have accidents involving themselves than other drivers in Britain and are more likely to have accidents on unfamiliar, poor congested roads abroad. Accidents in vehicles or on the road are one of the riskiest aspects of travel abroad. Yet most people worry far more about disease, which causes just 9% of deaths, or terrorism, which presents a negligible risk.
Falls are a common cause of injury abroad and are often associated with alcohol. They are particularly likely in older adults, due to poor vision, imbalance and postural hypotension. Walking barefoot or in sandals increases the risk of falls and foot injuries.

Advice for road users while abroad

Travellers should:

- insist on wearing a seat belt when in a car or coach.
- Check to see coach, bus, taxi or hire car is roadworthy and safe
- beware of driving in countries with poor traffic regulations such as Egypt and India
- avoid motorbikes as they are particularly dangerous - even in European countries such as Greece. If using one, wear a helmet
- be careful at night on poorly lit ,or poorly maintained roads
- be obsessively careful when crossing roads, as zebra crossings are often ignored
- avoid alcohol if deciding to drive, but be aware that locals may not do so and that alcohol may disturb balance and gait making a fall more likely.
- wear a helmet and safety jacket if using a bicycle.
- think of road safety

References

1.Ward D. Ocean Cruising 2005 Berlitz Pub. London.
2.McIntosh I Health risks for those going on sea cruises. 2006.. North European Travel Health Conference. Edinburgh
3.Wheeler R. Travel Health at Sea. Principles and Practice of Travel Med.2001 274-85 Ed Zuckerman J Wiley Chichester
4.McIntosh I. Elderly travellers. In Trav. Med and Migrant Health. Churchill Livingstone. Edinburgh1992 7.107-114
5.Internat. Passenger Survey 2003 HMSO London6.Polonev K/Characteristics of morbidity among passengers. Proceedings 4th. Internat. Conf. Marine Med. Varna 1972,298-303
7.Ulewitz K.1976.Epidemic on a passenger ship. Bull. Instit.Marit. Trop Med. 27.105-8
8.Baterman W. The ugly duckling, a different kind of ship. Can. Med. Assoc. J. 1990142.365-71
9 Travellers' Health,Chap 7 Centres for Disease contol and Prevention Atlanta 2005
10 Smith A. in Travellers Health Ed Dawood R. 4th. Edn. Oxford Univ. Press 2002.277-89
11.Davies J. Polar cruise ships travelling Antarctica and the Arctic Brit. Trav. Health Assoc J. 2006 7..48
12.Davies J.Antarctic tourism and its risks. Brit. Trav. Health Assoc J. 2006.7.35-8.
13 .Prociv P Health aspects of Antarctic tourism J Trav Med. 1998 4 210-21957-1993
14 .Dahl E. Anatomy of a world Cruise. J. Trav. Med6.168-71
15 Polonev K.Characteristics of morbidity among passengers. Proceedings 4th. Internat. Conf. Marine Med. Varna 1972,298-303
16 .British Travel Health Assoc. J Shipping News.2006 54-55
17 Peake D. Grey C. Ludwig MR Descriptive epidemioly of injury and illness among cruise ship passengers. Ann. Emerg. Med. 1999.33.67-72
18.Baterman W. The ugly duckling, a different kind of ship . Can. Med. Assoc. J. 1990142.365-71
19.Martinovic N Morbidity of passengers and crew Adriana Trav. Med .Internat.1997 15.194-199
20.Jareman B Problems of medical care on a passenger ship Bull Instit. Marit. Trop. Med.1988. 39.137-48,
21.Carter. Shipboard medicine on package cruises Brit. Med J. 1972 550-53
22.DiGiavanna T Rosa T Shipboard Med. Ann Emerg Med. 1993 10.1639
23 Dahl E.Passenger mortalities aboard cruise ship. Internat. Marit.Health.2001.519-3
24 Hudson Neilson P Dahl E. Factors associated with injuries aboard ships J. Trav. Med.2006 13.67-
25 Oliver . Health problems at Sea Practitioner 1977 21,202-10
26 McIntosh I. Health ,hazard and the higher risk traveller. Quay Books Mark Allan Pub Dinton 1993 23-34
27 Elbert h. 100 years of public health authority in Hamburg. Bull. Instit. Marit. Trop Med. 1992 43.5-11
28.McIntosh I Travel, trauma, risks and health promotion. Quay Books. Marl Allen Pub.Dinton. 1998 29.Minooee A. Rickman L Clin Inf Disease 1999,29,737-44.
30.Beyrer K Lai S Dreesman et al Legionnaires disease outbreak associated with a cruise ,liner Aug.2003. Govt. Instit of Public Health. Hannover Germany. Sept29.2006
31.Jernigan Doffman J. Certon MS. Et al Outbreak of Legionnaires disease among cruise ship passengers . Lancet 1996 347 494-99
32.Kura E.Ammemura J Yagita K. Outbreak of Legionnaires disease 2003 PMID 9876197. Pubmed.
33.Azara A Piana A Sotjui G et al BMC Public Health 2006 18.100
34. Quarantine div. Centres for Disease Control and prevention CDC1998a, 1998b.Mortlality and morbidity report. 47.638
35.Health Canada 1998.Influenza outbreak Canada Communicable disease report. 24.9-11
36 CDC(Quarantine div. Centres for Disease Control and Prevention.Guidelines.jan 28. 1999..
37 Quarantine div. Centres for Disease Control and prevention 1CDC 2000a.b. 2001.Report 50

References contd.

38 WHO Compendium of food and waterborne disease and Legionnaires disease associated with ships 1970-2000. 2002WHO/WHO/01.

39 Daniels N Neimann J Karpati A Travellers diarrhoea at sea
et al J Inf Dis 2000 181 1495

40.Koo D Maloney K Tauxe R epidemiology of diarrhoeal disease outbreaks on cruise ships 1986 –1993 JAMA 1996 275 545-7

41.Snyder J Wells JG. Ashuk J. outbreak of invasive E.Coli gastroenteritis on cruise ships Am J. Trop

42.Consumers Assoc.UK Cruise ship hygiene. Report 2005 Which.

43. McIntosh I Motion Sickness J.Trav. Med. 1998 5.89-91

44.Pingree B.JNM investigation into drugs for sea sickness.J. RN Med. Service. 1994 80.76-80

45 Brennan F. A guide to healthy cruising. Brit. Trav. Health Assoc.J. 2000 1, 17-20

46 McIntosh I.Pitstops and pitfalls- A health guide for older travellers Quay Pub.Mark Allan Pub. Salisbury.1996

47 McIntosh I Health and safety on Cruise ships Brit.Trav. Health Assoc. J. 2007 9.10-17
Iain B. McIntosh

48 Internat. Passenger Survey 2007/8/ Office Nat. Stats. London

Iain B.McIntosh

Chapter 6

Travel Induced Illness.

"Travel in the young is a part of education: in the old, part of experience."
Francis Bacon

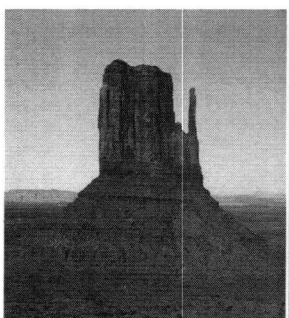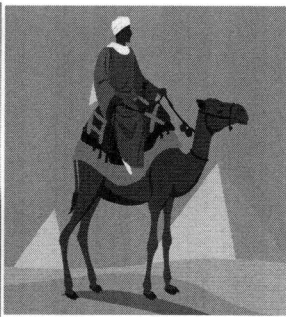

Travel to hot, arid, dry and humid places

The effects of travel related illness on older people are poorly recorded. One general practice based study of medical intervention for illness sustained abroad and its impact on over 65 year olds, showed that almost half became ill. Much was minor in nature and responded to self medication, but ill health often interfered with holiday plans and for some ruined the vacation. 1 Adventurous older people are exploring distant parts of the globe with hostile climates, which present a challenge to health.

Electrolyte and fluid imbalance

Poor control of fluid balance in elderly travellers can have an adverse effect on well-being, when they are exposed to high environmental temperatures. Body fluid regulation is critically affected by age- related changes in function of sweat glands and kidneys and in the sensation of thirst. Older people are more vulnerable in a very hot, arid, or humid environment than the young, due to increased frailty and disease load, but also to reduced efficiency of adaptive processes and control of fluid balance.

Increasing age brings decline in body mass – the percentage of water in the body in the old is lower than in young adults- and the decrease in intracellular volume is more marked than in extra cellular volume. Losing a litre of water has a proportionately greater adverse effect in the aged.2

Under heat stress, regulation of body fluids, depends upon kidney and sweat gland function and thirst sensation. Homeostasis is affected by intrinsic and extra renal control mechanisms. The ageing kidney exhibits detrimental anatomical and functional change over time. Renal mass is lost and there is decrease in renal blood flow, with an almost linear decline in glomerular filtration rate.3

Older people are more sensitive to water depletion. Attenuation of renal tubular activity results in impaired renal response to arginine vasopressin and elders are more sensitive to water depletion. They are also less responsive to the renin-angiotensin-aldosterone axis and have decreased plasma renin and aldosterone activity, which predisposes them to natriuresis and salt depletion. The decline in renal function also ensures they are less able to excrete a salt load, or to adjust to salt deficiency.

Even without the effects of renal disease the old are at greater risk of developing hyperkalaemia due to reduced kidney function and reduced ability to correct acid load.[4] Fluid deprivation, or restriction in a very hot environment, such as the tropics, can have a deleterious effect on the elderly traveller. In aged people, control systems for thirst and satiety are attenuated. There is a reduced sensation of thirst. They have a higher osmotic operating point for thirst awareness and a decreased response to unloading of baroreceptors by hypovolaemia.[5]Due to this lack of awareness, there is a higher risk of dehydration occurring. There is also marked atrophy of sweat glands with ageing and reduced neuro-humoural control. Diminished sweating capacity contributes to thermo-regulatory failure, compounded by impaired vasodilatation. Both water deficiency and salt-efficiency heat exhaustion occur in elderly people who exercise hard in conditions of heat extremes.

Dehydration is the most common fluid and electrolyte imbalance in old adults, with three elements:-

Isotonic dehydration involves a balanced loss of solutes and water, which occurs with severe vomiting or diarrhoea – common occurrences in world travellers.

Hypotonic dehydration occurs when sodium is lost at a greater rate than water, resulting in serum sodium concentration of less than 130mmols./litre

Hypertonic dehydration is where water losses exceed these of sodium, and serum sodium concentration is greater than 145 mmpl/litre .This can occur with fever or decreased water intake.

Hypernatraemic dehydration also often occurs in elderly people in very hot conditions, as an end result of heavy sweating as sweat is a hypotonic salt solution.

Co morbidity can increase the likelihood of illness from exposure to enduring heat and humidity extremes.[6] Drug medication can interfere with excretion of free water and diuretics have a high incidence of adverse effects on fluid balance. [7]Medical conditions which reduce cardiac and renal reserves can affect capacity to respond adequately to heat stressors. Chronic renal failure, the end point of diabetes mellitus, hypertension, renal sclerosis or obstruction and the tendency to slip into cardiac failure, are common conditions affecting elderly people. The afflicted easily move into critical water and fluid imbalance when exposed to heat stress.

Summary

Older people are vulnerable in a very hot, arid or humid environment due to :-
- increased frailty and disease load,
- reduced efficiency of adaptive processes and control of fluid balance
- increased sensitivity to water depletion
- less ability to excrete salt load, or to adjust to salt deficiency
- greater risk of developing hyperkalaemia
- reduced sensibility to sensation of thirst
- higher risk of dehydration
- diminished sweating capacity [8]

Identifying those at potential risk

Three groups of elderly people have been identified as at higher risk of developing heat exposure problems.

1 *Active people* fit enough to indulge in hard exercise, can incur significant water and electrolyte losses when pursuing strenuous physical activities in hot climates, particularly if these occur at high altitude.

2 *Sedentary elders* who are over-clothed, drink inadequate fluids fail to replace loss of salt, rely on an inadequate adaptive sweating capacity and vasodilatation to dissipate heat

3 *People with chronic conditions,* such as renal, or cardiac failure.

Symptoms of dehydration.

Classic symptoms of water depletion are :-

- fatigue,
- giddiness
- thirst with nausea,
- vomiting
- muscle cramps.

The condition may result in heat stroke and death. In predominant salt depletion, thirst is less marked, but fatigue is more prominent as is giddiness and vomiting, with potential death from oligaemic shock.

There are no pathognomonic signs, or symptoms. The most useful indicators are dry mouth, tongue and mucous membranes, sunken eyes, body weakness, and confusion, which are however common to other conditions in older people. Thirst is the main presentation in water deficiency, but less so with salt shortage. The volume of urine is low and concentrated.

Management

Those at high risk should be identified prior to global travel to very warm, humid areas. Diabetics particularly and those with thyroid disease should be targeted.

Potential elderly travellers need advice on risk and preventive measures

Ensuring appropriate fluid intake and reducing insensible heat loss by behavioural precautions are important, to maintain adequate fluid balance.

Light fabric, loose fitting clothing of light colour should be worn.

Adjustments in medications such as diuretics may be necessary

Adequate fluid and salt intake is vital with a recommended daily intake of fluid of 1600 mls. per 70Kg of weight in 24 hours, enhanced in hot, dry temperatures overseas 8

Salt supplementation will be appropriate for physically hyperactive old folk, especially those on high treks or desert and jungle safari.9Attention should be drawn to the health hazard of physical over-activity in heat extremes.

The need to carry water and check for indicators of possible fluid imbalance must be emphasised in pretravel consultation.

Conclusion

Fluid and electrolyte imbalance can affect elderly travellers to hot climatic regions,

Reduction in efficiency of renal water and electrolyte regulation, sweating function and thirst sensation make older travellers a higher risk group.

Water and salt deficiency heat exhaustion can lead to oligaemia and heat stroke in old travellers

Intense physical activity in hot, arid and humid conditions is likely to promote water deficiency in the old.

Pre-existing cardiac and renal disorders increase the risk of fluid imbalance,

At-risk world travellers should be identified prior to travel and advised of the risk and appropriate precautions to minimise it.

Gastrointestinal illness (acute gastrointestinal enteritis (AGE)accounted for half of all reported illness with heart and skin conditions in second place. Cardiac problems often resulted in hospitalisation .10% successfully self treated. 18% sought medical consultation and a visit from a doctor while abroad. 8% were hospitalised because of travel induced illness and 11% were ill enough to seek consultation with a doctor on return home. 10Some of this infective illness was preventable and might have been avoided by good pretravel advice and precautions.

Surveillance of 14,227 air travellers of all ages returning to Scotland from abroad revealed 37% were affected by illness.10 Alimentary symptoms accounted for 76% of symptoms. Older travellers may be more adversely affected by AGE if they become dehydrated and lose electrolyte balance.11

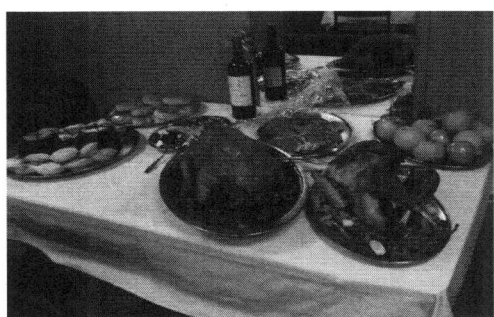

Infection Risk-Travel Related Diarrhoea

Travel related diarrhoea (TRD) is usually the result of ingestion of infected food or water and defined as three or more unformed stools in 24 hours, with one associated enteric symptom of, abdominal pain, cramps, vomiting, fever, or tenesmus. Often with sudden onset acute diarrhoea, no invasive pathogen can be identified and fluid and electrolyte disturbance is not a major concern. The clinical syndrome can by different organisms.

- Enterotoxigenic E.Coli ETEC) is most common
- Campylobacter,
- Salmonella
- rotovirus
- norovirus.

Some cases develop into dysentery- diarrhoea containing blood -usually caused by shigella dysenteriae, or entamoeba hystolytica – an important management distinction 12

(TRD) is the predominant travel associated illness, with prevalence rates varying from 8% to 50% depending on country visited 13.14.15

- World travellers are 6.5 times more likely to experience TRD than if they had stayed at home 10
- Three levels of risk for TRD are identified with intermediate incidence rates occurring in destinations in the Caribbean, Southern Europe, Israel and Japan and South Africa and high rates between 20 and 55% in developing parts of the world.16

- rates of 20-55% occur in developing parts of the world.[16]

Symptoms of TRD

Diarrhoea frequently starts two to three days after exposure to infection, or a new environment.A second episode often commences a week later. Untreated the condition lasts about 4 days, with 1% of the affected suffering symptoms for a month 6 In the very old, associated dehydration and loss of body salts may endanger life.

Management

Two thirds of sufferers choose to treat their diarrhoea, with half self- medicating and the others seeking professional prescription.[2]

Anti-motility agents are available as over the counter (OTC) pharmacy products and are used widely without adverse effect. TRD could be avoided if the traveller abstained from consumption of contaminated food and water and was scrupulous with personal hygiene in hand washing, after toilet and food contact. Codeine preparations are commonly used by travellers as anti-diarrhoeal remedies [7]

Loperamide, an anti-motility agent, can be considered the anti-diarrhoeal of choice for symptomatic treatment. [16,17,18,19] Placebo studies show antimotility agents to be fast acting and clinically effective in mild to moderate, non-invasive diarrhoea[20]They are safe and effective when used in non-dysenteric diarrhoea [21,22,23]. They relieve acute intestinal spasm, abdominal pain and distension, common symptoms of acute diarrhoea. Loperamide is a peripherally acting opiate without abuse potential, which does not cross the blood-brain barrier and has little impact on the systemic circulation due to its mainly liver and faecal excretion. A therapeutic 4mg. dose of loperamide in a healthy adult does not slow orocaecal transit and in diarrhoea states will normalise transit [17] There was no prolongation of illness or complication if these drugs were administered in cases of diarrhoea, where invasive organisms were identified, when used with antimicrobials.[24,25] These drugs will reduce the number of unformed stools and shorten the duration of symptoms. When compared to the antimicrobial medication alone, they do not prolong fever or delay pathogen excretion in stools.

Many elderly people take other routine medications and possible drug interactions must be considered before prescription.Loperamide may mask dehydration and depletion of electrolytes. Dehydration may increase the variability of response to the drug.

The early use of this medication may be indicated in older travellers. Delay in active treatment intervention is difficult to justify. [26]An appropriate prescription can bring travellers prompt relief and diminish risk from dehydration.

Use of loperamide and an antimicrobial brings fastest relief with quinolones, cotrimoxizole and doxycycline all effective. Quinilones work in single, two and three dose regimens and prolonged medication is unnecessary.

Oral replacement therapy *(ORT) must be* considered for the frail elderly as they are at higher risk from dehydration.[27] Ageing is associated with reduction in beneficial colonic bifidobacteria. Galacto-oligosaccharides (GOS) stimulate growth of bifidobacteria .A comparative study using a second generation prebiotic GOS mixture (B-GOS) showed significant increase in beneficial bifidobacteria and decrease in less beneficial colonic cells, increase of phagocytosis, natural killer cell activity and production of anti-inflammatory cytokynin interleukin-10 .Dietary B-Gos supplementation in healthy elderly people may result in positive effects on both microflora composition and immune response. Older world travellers may benefit from a 7 day pretravel and vacation dietary complement of B-GOS

Conclusion

Pre-travel advice regarding traveller's diarrhoea can help reduce the duration of the illness. [28]
Patients should be encouraged carry OTC medications such as loperamide and self treat simple acute episodes of TRD.[29]
Use of an antimotility agent and an antibacterial brings fastest relief.
ORT should be considered as dehydration can present early in older people with acute diarrhoea.[30]

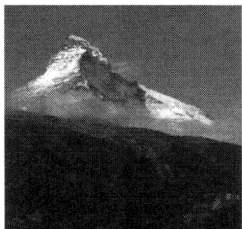

High Altitude Effects

High Altitude Illness

Many older people are adventurous and participate in holiday packages which can expose them to high altitude environments. Several of the world's airports such as La Paz and Cusco are 3,000m. above sea-level and arriving passengers can succumb to altitude illness on arrival,. Standard tours across Chile, Bolivia, Peru, the Andes and the North American Rockies can bring high altitude illness, One of my patients developed Acute Mountain Sickness in a taxi crossing the high mountain pass between Marrakesh and the Sahara. Himalayan tours are popular with no age exclusions and travellers frequently get altitude sickness on walking treks in Nepal and Bhutan. Many tourists including the elderly are unaware of the health risk they run by exposure to high altitude.
This can induce illness from acute mountain sickness.The partial pressure of oxygen in the atmosphere diminishes with increasing altitude.Older people with diminished lung cpacity and function (see Chap.1) when exposee to lack of oxygen are more are disadvantaged compared to the young .they are also vulnerable to complications of exposure to increasing altitude. Travellers living at high altitude can experience headaches, breathlessness, sleeping badly and loss of appetite. These are symptoms of AMS (acute mountain sickness).-an uncomfortable but not life threatening condition. If symptoms become severe and increase in altitude continues, an increase of fluid in the brain (High Altitude Cerebral Oedema - HACE), or fluid in the lungs (High Altitude Pulmonary Oedema - HAPE) can happen and these conditions can kill quickly. Older people are also at greater risk of stroke and retinal artery occlusion due to the increase in viscosity in the blood which occurs with altitude. Altitude starts to have an effect between 1,500 - 2,000m. The body tries to make up for the change in oxygen levels over a few days of exposure.
Given enough time to adapt, most people can adjust to altitudes up to about 5,000m (Everest base camp).The body slowly adapts to lower oxygen levels –acclimatisation-but different people acclimatise at different speeds Ascending too fast to above 2,500m and maintained, or increased altitude thereafter exposes the individual to altitude illnesses which are common There are no indicators to indicate those at high risk with first exposure to a high altitude environment however if an individual has suffered symptoms on previous exposure, they are more likely to experience them on further exposure.(See Chap.14)

Symptoms
- Headache.
- Nausea
- Vomiting.
- Fatigue
- Poor appetite .
- Dizziness.
- Sleep disturbance.

Dehydration the most common fluid and electrolyte imbalance in old adults as has been mentioned previously can also add to the risk from AMS. High altitude environment are often very dry and water sources limited, Strenuous activity, over-heating and inadequate fluid intake makes dehydration a significant risk for those who travel high.

Management Guidelines.

Pretravel precautionary advice is important with instructions to:-
Travel slowly, over 3,000m,
Sleep no more than 300m higher than previous night at the end of each day.(Going higher is possible there is decent to lower level to sleep each night , sleep ("walk high- sleep low"). If impracticable and descent is not possible,organising a rest day before further ascent allows body time to 'catch-up'.
Consider use of a carbonic anhydrase inhibitor prior to entering this environment.
Acetazolamide (Diamox) can be used to reduce the effects of AMS and is useful where large height gains are unavoidable. It does have side effects of sudden paraethesia in limbs and increases risk from dehydration.
Use a simple scorecard to measure disturbance to normal breathing and sleeping and question whether are symptoms getting better or worse?
If symptoms worsen, descent is obligatory.- to at least 500 to 1,000m lower level for sleeping).
Give the body extra time to acclimatise.
Maintain a high fluid input to avoid dehydration.

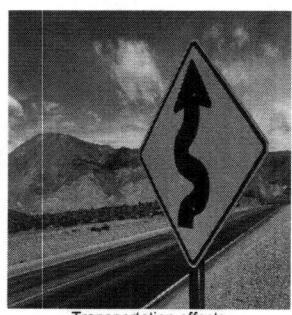
Transportation effects

Motion sickness (kinetosis), occurs where there is disagreement between visually perceived movement and the vestibular system's sense of movement.

This can occur on any form of transport with most people affected on ships and small boats, in cars and coaches. Dizziness, fatigue, and nausea are the most common symptoms of motion sickness About 33% of people are susceptible to motion sickness even in mild circumstances such as being on a boat in calm water, although nearly 66% of people are susceptible in more severe conditionsElderly people are no more susceptible than the young but prolonged vomiting can bring electrolyte disturbance and dehydration with more serious consequences in older people. Antiemetic medication can also interact or interfere with routine medication.

Seasickness

100% of ship passengers can suffer in rough conditions, particularly in Southern Ocean and Drake Passage. Most cruise ships however have stabilizers which diminishes roll and reduces the number as affected passengers. Cabins at the centre of the ship display least vertical acceleration.(See Chap.5)

Vehicle sickness. The effect is worst when looking down and is significantly lessened by looking forward and outside of a land vehicle.The front seat of a car, forward coaches of a train, upper or wing seats in a plane may give u a smoother ride. Looking out of car or coach into the distance can reduce effects and reading aboard is best avoided.

Medication Prophylactic medicaments should be taken an hour or two prior to exposure to the unstable environment.Favoured drugs are cinnarizine, scopolamine and promethazine. Scopolamine was more effective than cinnarizine, but in mild motion cinnarizine was better tolerated.

Psychological Illness.

Britons face travel over, under or across the sea when undertaking travel abroad . Air, land and sea transit creates anxiety in older travellers. Slowing of mental response to stimuli and central processing information and slower reaction to cognitive tasks in old age makes them more vulnerable to the stressors now inseparable from global relocation.[30] Passage to and through air terminals ,rail termini and sea ports has become more stressful and anxiety provoking. There are concerns about the mechanical safety of aeroplanes and rational fears of hijack, terrorist attack, and the physiological effects of prolonged travel on the venous circulation.(see Chap.9)

Many older people find conventional travel modes and translocation moderately or severely stressful, with many fearful and some phobic of travel Anxiety generated by relocation and transportation is associated with travel fatigue which can last for a day or two after arrival[31]The increase in heart rate and blood pressure associated with the anxiety of airport transit may only discomfit a fit traveller but can be disadvantageous in older people. In those with cardiac problems this may precipitate arrhythmia, myocardial infarction and stroke [32] Terrorist attacks of 2001 brought a disproportionate public psychological response in that, many potential travellers gave up flying and took alternative transport. Analysis of fatal accidents showed the number of Americans who lost lives driving on roads, to avoid flying, was higher than all those killed on affected flights .Their behavioral response was disproportionate to the actual personal risk of flying. This risk misperception with change in behaviour provokes unnecessary and inappropriate anxiety .Worries about developing deep vein thrombosis with prolonged flying are common, with the public relatively well informed about risk, but poor in risk assessment. The disproportionate reaction to dread risk events merits reconditioning of the individual and education in risk assessment.[33,34,35]

Health professionals working in the travel health scene should be aware of the psychological effects of relocation and transit and the risk to the wellbeing of older and vulnerable people embarking on international travel. They deserve risk assessment before departure, information on potential health challenge, education regarding misperceptions and encouragement to take measures to minimise threat. They should be identified and offered counselling and treatment .Appropriate advice and improved preplanning could diminish the impact of many travel induced stressors.

Management

Provision of informative facts on actual risk and dread risk and correction of misperceptions

Recommended preplanning of travel programme

Recommended precautions eg deep vein thrombosis

Advice on available therapy (eg panic states and phobias)

References.

1 McIntosh I Power K . Travel induced illness in the elderly 1991 Scot. Med. 11. 4.14-15

2 Allison S. Lobo D. Fluid and electrolytes in the elderly . Curr. Opin. Clin. Nutr Metab Care 2004 .27-33

3 Lye M. Disturbances of homeostasis in Tallis FC (Ed) Geriatric Med. and Geront. 5th Ed. London Churchill Livingstone 1998 925-48

4 Biswas K Mulkerrin E Potassium homeostasis in the elderly QJ Med 1997 90. 487-92

5 Kenney W Chiu P Influence of age on thirst and fluid intake Med. Sc. Sports Exercise 2001 33. 1524-32

6 Gurwitz J Field T et al Incidence and preventability of adverse drug events among older persons in the ambulatory sweating. JAMA 2003 289. 1107-1

7 Schwartz J Who is sensitive to extremes of temperature. Epidemiol. 2005 16 61-7

8 Collins K Fluid balance of elderly people in hot environments. Geriatric Med. 2009. ….385-90

9 Department of Health . Heat wave plan for England. Dept of Health 2005

10 Cossar J. Review of travel associated illness 1988 Trav. Med.50-54Springer-Verlag 6 London

11.McIntosh I. Travel in the elderly 1992 .Chap 7. Quay Books . Lancaster.

12 Steffen R. Lobel H. Traveller's Diarrhoea. J. Wilderness Med. 1994.5.56-66

13. Porter JD. Travelling hopefully, returning ill. British Medical Journal 1992 304 1323-4

14. Gorbach SL, Peltolah H Textbook of Travel Medicine and Health.1997, (Eds. R Steffen and H DuPont). Becker Publications, Hamilton, Ontario.

15 Reed J. McIntosh I. Power K. Travel Illness and the Family Practitioner. Journal of Travel Medicine 1994, 1.192-7

16. Farthing M. Traveller's Diarrhoea. Gut. 1994, 35: 1-4

17 Fletcher P. Benefit/risk considerations with respect to OTC de-scheduling of loperamide. Arzneim Forsch 1995, 45: 608-13

18. Gorbach SL Treating diarrhoea. (Editorial) British Medical Journal1997, 314: 1776-7

19. DuPont HNL. Guidelines on acute infectious diarrhoea in adults.American Journal of Gastroenterology.1997; 92 :1962-75

20 Kaplan M. Priore M et al A multicentre controlled trial of a liquid loperamide product versus placebo in the treatment of acute diarrhoea in children. 1999 Clin. Paediatrics 38.579-91

21 Johnson PC. Comparison of loperamide with bismuth subsalicylate for the treatment of acute traveller's diarrhoea. J.Amer. Med. Assoc. 1986255.757-60

22. Ericsson, CD Johnson PC. Safety and efficacy of loperamide. American. Journal of Medicine. 1990, 88:10-14S

23.Steffen R. Efficacy and side effects of 6 agents in the treatment of travellers diarrhoea. Travel Medicine International. 1988, 153-7

24 Van Loon FPL. Double blind trial of loperamide for treating acute watery diarrhoea in expatriots in Bangladesh. Gut. 1989, 30: 492-5

25 .Murphy GS. Ciprofloxacin and loperamide in the treatment of bacillary dysentery. Annals of Internal Medicine. 1993, 118: 582-

26 Schiller LR, Santa Ana CA, Morawski SG, et al. Mechanism of the antidiarrheal effect of loperamide. Gastroenterol. 1984; 86: 1475-83.

27 Wingate D. Phillips S. Lewis S et al Guidelines for adults on self medication for the treatment of acute diarrhoea. 2001 Aliment. Pharmacol.Ther. 15.773-82

28 Swanson V. McIntosh I. Howell K. A study of gp's attitudes to acute diarrhoea management. Scot. Med. 1999.18.6-7

29 McIntosh I.Reed JM, Power K Travellers diarrhoea and the effect of pre-travel health advice in general practice. British Journal of General Practice, 1997, 47, 71-75.

30 Gurcharan SR Essentials of Geriatric Medicine 2010 2nd.Ed. Radcliffe Pub London.

31Waterhouse J Reilly T. Edwards B J Sports Science 2004 (10) 946-65

32 DeHart R Health issues of air travel. Ann Rev Public Health 003 24 133-51Bracewell C Gray R

33 Gikerenzer G. Dread risk, Sept 11 and fatal accident Psychol. Sc. 2004 15 286-7

34 Gauld J. McIntosh I .Attitudes to travel after terrorist events of 2001. 2002 .BTHA J .3 62-7

35 Swanson V McIntosh I Perceived threats to life and limb and effects of anxiety provoking events on the traveller. BTHA J 2004 5 48-52

Chapter 7

The cardiac and diabetic traveller

Knowledge of the world can only be acquired in the world and not in a closet. Lord Chesterfield

Environmental factors ensure that global travellers experience higher morbidity and mortality rates than if they had stayed at home. Pre-existing conditions such as cardiovascular disease, chronic obstructive airways disease and diabetes mellitus also play a prominent role in morbidity and mortality statistics for travellers, particularly among older age groups.

Causes of death in travellers while abroad [1]

Cause	%
Cardiovascular Disease	49.0
Medical,non- cancerous conditions	13.7
Trauma	22.0
Cancer	5.9
Other conditions	5.5
Suicide/Homicide	2.9
Infectious disease	1.0

Cardiac events

Cardiovascular events cause about 50% of deaths during air travel and are the second most frequent reason for evacuation. Several factors increase the risk of a cardiac event en route and at the overseas destination. Physiological and psychological pressures on travellers have increased in the last decade due to incremental changes in security and additional terrorist threat at airports, rail termini and ferry ports. Air and land traffic congestion and new environmental and climatic factors create delay, hassle and uncertainty which can push vulnerable individuals from physiological stability into systems failure. Inability to meet cardiac demands and respiratory and metabolic distress may become life threatening, at a time when immediacy of available emergency care may not equate with that of the home environment .The inadequacies of travel health insurance can also be exposed at this time of medical need. Insurers can only provide the best medical evacuation resources available in the local milieu. Optimal care cannot be provided in transit locations such as an aircraft and in many tourist vacation destinations around the world.

Travel to departure point.

Anxieties and stresses about leaving home, reaching the airport, transport and new location develop, as departure day nears and heighten as the traveller leaves home .Time constraints and deadlines bring adrenaline rush and psychological arousal. Unaccustomed physical demands such as hauling luggage, long walkways and the hassle of transfers from station to air or sea port, add to in-transit stressors. A fit health older individual may cope with these challenges, but the burden may push those with a pre-existing medical condition into respiratory or cardiac failure, or precipitate myocardial and cerebrovascular ischaemia and infarction. The risk increases with prolongation of travel due to transport delay- a common feature of modern travel.

Air travel

This transport mode can bring arterial oxygen desaturation with change in cabin pressurisation, along with forced immobility and potential dehydration. These effects can induce;-

- Chest pain and angina

- Dyspnoea and pulmonary oedema

- Cardiac arrhythmia

- Venous constriction and deep vein thrombosis

The Air Traveller with Heart Disease. The older traveller with existing cardiac ischaemia, angina and heart rhythm irregularities may find their symptoms exacerbated in the cabin environment.Those with pacemakers and cardio converters may experience problems with security scanners.[2]

Travellers with heart disease should:-

- Plan the journey by land and air as carefully as they choose their vacation hotel or ship cabin

- Purchase comprehensive travel insurance

- Acquire pneumococcal immunisation and annual influenza immunisation

- Choose antimalarial and an-emetic drugs, with due regard to contraindications and drug interactions

- Consider use of executive airport transfer lounges to diminish airport stress

- Consider travel in an upper class cabin for a less stressful flying experience.

Advice for traveller preparing for a long flight

Advise airline in advance of travel via the Passenger Medical Clearance Unit. Complete Medical Information Form [MEDIF] and Travellers' Medical Card [FREMEC for frequent travellers] for stable, non- progressive, chronic conditions. The airline will wish to confirm that the potential traveller can walk 100 m on the flat, at a normal pace without severe breathlessness.[3]

Notify airline in advance of need for:-

Porter, electric buggy, wheelchair and airport oxygen.Not all airlines supply oxygen at take-off & landing. Oxygen must be booked in advance (portable cylinder, fixed rate of 2-4 L/min by Hudson mask/nasal cannula) Oxygen concentrators are available (concentrate oxygen in ambient air by removing nitrogen) British Airways & United airlines charge £50-£100, other lines the price of another seat (£55 to £550).Virgin airline currently makes no charge: economy & premium economy class. For upper class passengers there may be no facility for oxygen for take- off & landing, as the oxygen cylinder cannot be stowed safely [4]

On the flight

* Support stockings should be worn –applied before leaving home.

* Warfarin can be continued as normal.

* Diuretic medication should be taken as usual

* Drug medication must be carried in hand luggage in adequate amount

* Exercise limbs. Walk about the aircraft if possible

Adequate Non-alcoholic non-carbonated fluids should be taken in flight

Contra-indications to flying and duration of estriction [1,5]

* Uncomplicated myocardial infarction -7 days–if complicated MI => 4 to 6 weeks

* Severe or non-stabilised heart failure

* Unstable angina

* CABG procedure, Open heart surgery => 10-14 days

* Angioplasty, Stent => 3 -5 days

* Uncontrolled cardiac arrhythmias

* Uncontrolled Hypertension

* Severe symptomatic valvular heart disease

Contraindications contd.

- Implantable cardioverter defibrillator (ICD): Prohibition on flying when ICD has delivered a shock, until condition considered stable.1

- Pacemaker or ICD insertion: flying acceptable after 2 days. If pneumothorax at insertion: flight possible after 2 wks.1

- Post ablation intervention: flight acceptable after 2 days but there is increased risk risk of VTE.1

Other Contra-indications to flying

- Acute Deep Vein Thrombosis –no flying until patient is stabilised on anticoagulants

- Cerebrovascular accident – if uncomplicated, individual may fly within 3 days (clearance is needed if travelling within 10 days)

- Brain surgery -10 days no flying after event

- Generalised seizure –24 hours delay before flight after occurrence

- Subarachnoid haemorrhage-10 days delay before flight Departure Security clearance.

- Predeparture Security Clearance

- Stent, mechanical valve in place. The passenger can safely walk through security machines, as these will not trigger an alarm

- Pacemaker/ICD: metal casings may trigger alarm. The hand-held metal detector should be requested and the operator advised not to place it directly over the pacemaker, or repeatedly sweep over device

The Traveller with Heart Disease who becomes ill while abroad

Consideration should be given to stopping prescribed diuretics and Ace inhibitors and seeking specialist advice if there is severe vomiting, diarrhoea, dehydration, hypotension, oliguria, 3kg weight loss , pulmonary or peripheral oedema.

Air Travellers and peripheral vascular disease

Air travel bring s increased risk in elderly people from venous thromboembolism (VTE)–Risk increases1 when flight > 4 hours with risk peaking at $\geq$ 8 hours flight duration .6

Factors increasing risk for VTE:

•immobilisation (found in 75% of cases, with higher risk in non-aisle seating)

•dehydration, due to haemoconcentration and hyperviscosity of blood

•hypobaric hypoxia also:-

- recent surgery

- obesity also:-

- malignancy

- thrombophilia

- past VTE

VTE precautions

Support stockings (but not if existing peripheral arterial disease- PAD). Below knee hosiery should be fitted to the individual 'Activa', 'Flight', 'Mediven'brands are available and should be applied with the leg elevated or at least horizontal, prior to home departure.

Aspirin 75-300 mg is no longer advised, as side effects may outweigh the benefits of use .Aspirin has only been shown to be efficacious in arterial blood research.

<u>Passengers at high risk of VTE[1]</u>:

Passengers with thrombophilia, recurrent DVT, polycythaemia, Factor V Leiden, antithrombin deficiency, malignancy, POP on lower limbs, gross obesity, surgery lasting >30 min in the previous four weeks are at higher risk A recommended precaution is the prescription of LWMH e.g. dalteparin (Fragmin®) 2,500 -5,000u SC before outward and return flights.[2.6]

Passengers on Warfarin medication may need alteration in routine administration with long flights and transmeridian travel.

Case Example

If a traveller on warfarin is flying directly to Tokyo from London (11½ hour flight, 8 hour time difference). The first regular dose of warfarin on that day needs to be changed.4The individual will be exposed to changes in diet bringing change in gut flora and possible vitamin K balance . INR changes are likely with possible increase in alcohol input which can increase the INR. With change in the environment–at altitude > 2,400 m, (7,900 feet) aircraft cabin pressure there is a 2.7-fold increased risk for INR values to fall below target (effect of hypoxia on coagulation and drug metabolism.[7]

In a crossing of more than 6 time zones from the UK eg travel from Britain to mid-USA or East India) The First regular dose of warfarin for the day needs adjustment

In travel:-

WEST => increase dose by quarter, as the traveller is facing a longer day.

EAST => decrease dose by about one third.

The INR should be repeated after 2 weeks of stay at the destination.

Other problems for the traveller with heart disease

Photosensitivity from various drugs such as thiazides, doxycycline, amiodarone

Anxiety generated by stressors inseparable from global travel, may merit use of a beta-blocker

Paroxysmal supraventricular tachycardia can be precipitated by physiological or psychological stress. This can be terminated with reflex vagal stimulation, Valsalva manoeuvre, carotid sinus massage, by plunging the face into ice cold water or taking large sips of ice cold water. If recurrent, medication such as beta-blocker plus verapamil may be required.

The Diabetic Traveller

The diabetic traveller faces several problems in world travel relating to diet and medication. Cultural changes in eating and diet habit at the destination may require change in caloric intake and adjustment in medication. The crossing of time zones and restricted meal content and times may upset the metabolic balance. Adverse temperatures and the risk of hypothermia and hypothermia can result in morbidity in the diabetic and failure to protect insulin and maintain adequate personal stores of other diabetic drugs can be hazardous. Prescribed drugs to combat the condition may not be available at the destination or not be equivalent in dose and efficacy. It is vital that diabetic potential global travellers prepare for the journey well in advance and seek advice from family doctor, consultant physician and travel clinic staff before embarking on international trips to developing and remote countries.

Neither diabetics nor their medical advisers should regard diabetes as a contraindication to travel, but many problems may arise for diabetics during travel, including loss of diabetic control, travel-related infections, management of diabetic emergencies and practical problems of carrying and storing insulin, other supplies and equipment.

Pre-travel arrangements 8.9

The travel health professional should consider with the traveller-

All recommended vaccinations. These may give a temporary rise of blood sugar

Malaria chemoprophylaxis and insect repellents

Travel insurance (full declaration of clinical status required) -Diabetes UK

European Health Insurance Card

MedicAlert®identificaton bracelet.

Adequate and correct medication, glucose testing equipment, glucose tablets, syringes/needles, needle disposal container.

Glucagon to be administered by travelling companion/stewardess) GlucoGel (Hypostopgel) with written professional declaration of medical need for needles, syringes, pens, vials, monitoring devices and a NHS 'Repeat Prescription' form.

The Diabetic Potential Traveller should remember:-

- Insulin needs to be kept from freezing and protected from sunlight. For long travel and use in hot/cold regions: use of a wide-necked vacuum flask (rinse with cold water or ice daily) or insulated storage bag Special insulin wallets can be used on the aircraft with no need for refrigeration and should be carried in hand luggage.

- To carry on the person:- testing strips, glucometers.(In very hot/cold climate strips may over/under read.)

During travel:-

Anticipate delays, the freezing of insulin supplies in hold and lost luggage –need to carry emergency snacks –insulin/food and travel sickness medication

All medication, testing equipment, lancets –capped-and glucometer should be carried in hand luggage

Exercise limbs, walk about train and aircraft to mobilise limb muscles

Stockings for leg support should be applied to limbs before home departure.

Comfortable shoes or slippers should be worn on aeroplane, train or long distance coach

Avoid alcohol in transit

Tight glycaemic control during air travel is not necessary, but avoid hypoglycaemia

The Diabetic Traveller on insulin

A type 1 Diabetic patient, on insulin, is travelling to California (13hour flight, 8 hour difference, 9 time zones). The total dose of insulin needs to change by 2-4% per time zone crossed.

Should there be an increase or decrease in the total dose?

Travel up to 8 hours–stay on 'home time' for meals and injections

North ↔ South travel=> no change

Travel over8 hours (> 6 time zones)–adjust dose of insulin by 2-4% per time zone crossed (~ ⅓ of daily dose-2)5

East North -South West travel .

Insulin *(more than once daily)dose*

Monitor blood glucose frequently in-flight and accept there will be a relative hyperglycaemia In

westbound travel (longer day)–increase time between injections twice, by 2 to 3 hours each time.Increase insulin daily dose by 2-4% for each hour of time shift In Eastbound travel (shorter day), shorten time between injections. Decrease daily dose of insulin by 2-4% for each hour of time shift (~ ⅓ of daily dose)6.

Westbound travel (longer day)

If on a single dose, take usual dose on day of departure. On twice daily dose regimen take usual dose on day of departure then another 18 hours after am dose, but if blood glucose is greater than 13 mmol/l, take ⅓ of usual am. dose followed by a snack or meal, then usual morning dose at destination.

Eastbound travel (shorter day)

For single dose or twice daily (10-12-hourly dose) take Usual dose on day of departure. In Morning at destination: ⅔ of usual dose–10 h after am. dose. If glucose >13 mmol/l => take remaining ⅓ of usual dose followed by a snack or meal (if on twice daily dose regimen add this ⅓ to pm. dose).On second da take usual dose

Insulin & Airport Security

Carry a Prescription that matches the patient name & insulin in the box & label

GlucoGel & Glucagon-carry a prescription with matching name

Ask for hand-inspection of the insulin but Insulin can safely pass through X-rays .However insulin stability may be affected by remaining in the path of XRs longer than normal or if it is repeatedly exposed to X-rays

Carry insulin glucagen and glucogel only in checked baggage. Baggage stored in cargo subject to powerful X-rays and–severe changes in pressure and temperature

The Diabetic Traveller on oral hypoglycaemics

Stay on 'home time' for meals and medication

Adjust on arrival. Sulphonylurea dosages -may need to be altered to avoid hypoglycaemia

Carry glucose tablets

At destination

Some countries only have insulin U-40 or U-80 strengths therefore take an adequate supply

Adjust dose of insulin if undertaking –increased activity, overeating or less active than normal

Hot climates lead to increased absorption of insulin bringing risk of relative hypoglycaemia (dose may need to be reduced)

Travel to areas of high altitude: can cause insulin to expand and contract causing air pockets within the cartridge or pen

Practice a few "air shots" to ensure absence of air bubbles before injecting. Alternatively, revert to using a syringe and needle -it is usually possible to draw insulin out of a cartridge

Avoid walking barefooted on beach or at poolside to avoid laceration and infection

If traveller's diarrhoea occurs ,do not stop insulin or tablets, monitor glucose frequently, adjust insulin dose accordingly, .Hydrate and correct caloric input with carbohydrate-containing salt/sugar solution(8 level teaspoonfuls of sugar in 1 litre of safe water)

References.

1 Causes of Mortality in Travellers Hargarten et al. Ann Emergency Med 20:622-626, 1991

2 Cardiac devices1. Smith D et al. Fitness to fly for passengers with cardiovascular disease. Heart 2010;96:ii1-i6. doi:10.1136/hrt.2010.2030911.

3. McCarthy A. Chapter 24 in Keystone et al. Travel Medicine. 2nd edition, Mosby Elsevier 1.

4 http://www.britishairways.com/health/docs/before/airtravel_guide.pdf

5 Cannegieter SC et al. Travel-related venous thrombosis: results from a large population-based case control study (MEGA). PLoS Med 2006;3:e307

6 Schwarz T et al. Venous thrombosis after long-hall flights. Arch Intern Med 2003;163:2759-64

7 The Traveller on Warfarin1Ringwald J, et al. Travel and oral anticoagulation. J Travel Med 2009;volume 16, issue 4:276-283

8 Sane T et al. Travel related morbidity in travellers with diabetes Br Med J 1990;301:421

9 The Diabetic Traveller. Adapted from Benson E, Metz R. Management of diabetes during intercontinental travel. Bull Mason Clinic 1984-85;38:145-151 Practice Nursing 13(6): 259 - 262 (Jun 2002

Patient Information leaflet.

Tips for diabetic traveller

Plan ahead and consider the proposed trip activities and destination

Visit GP or diabetic advisor early to organises immunisations supplies and equipment -

Acquire a letter from GP. confirming diabetic status, and need for needles ,

Get a prescription for medication for longer than the trip schedule

Acquire diabetic identity bracelet and list of medications for emergency situations. Take copies of prescriptions & pharmacy contact information.

Carry pharmacist contact information and copies of prescriptions which will expedite replacement or ordering of medications and supplies while abroad but be aware that exact replacements of drugs and equipment may not be available.

Insurance should be organised on booking recording diabetes as a pre-existing condition. (Diabetes UK – can assist with appropriate policy)

Acquire and check validity of EHIC travelling within Europe.

Travelling by air "diabetic meals" may not be most appropriate. Check carbohydrate intake regularly and, if required, top-up with snacks en route.

Keep insulin on person at all times or carried in hand luggage, out of direct sunlight or freezing conditions - such as an aeroplane hold! If insulin comes in U-100 check the conversion rate in countries where it comes in U-40 or U-80 Travel to tropical regions of the world will require the keeping of insulin in a cold pack, or in a cool place,

Heat will affect the rate at which insulin is absorbed. In a high heat environment , insulin is absorbed quicker. It is important to monitor blood levels in hot weather and adjust diet as required.

In a cold climate insulin is absorbed slower.. Monitor blood sugar levels in extreme conditions and never insulin freeze.

Adjust insulin times on reaching destination

When travelling WEST lengthen the gap between insulin doses or add extra food with an extra dose until adjusted. When travelling EAST shorten the gap and reduce dosages. Check blood sugar regularly when crossing time zones, to determine need to adjust dosages. Perfect control might not be possible initially .

At Destination

Anticipate Traveller's diarrhoea and careful attention should be given to food and water ingestion. It is important to monitor blood sugar levels carefully if vomiting and diarrhoea occur. sick. Maintain a good level of carbohydrate content in diet. Seek medical advice if the problem continues beyond a few days. DiabeticTravel.co.uk specialises in Travel Insurance for Diabetics.

•   Airport security or immigration may request medication information. Traveling with an insulin pump can be difficult if you are unfamiliar with how to adjust them as you change time zones. Check with your doctor before traveling to determine the proper routine

In hand luggage, have a spare blood test machine, spare sensors, spare insulin and spare insulin pens.

If on an insulin pump, take spare reservoirs, infusion sets, an inserter, a bottle (or bottles) of insulin as well as some spare pump batteries. Traveling by car, coach or train, assume travel will extend over one additional day. If traveling by air, assume three additional days.

Carry a readily accessible medical history in case of hospitalisation .Include name and contact information of the home physician and family emergency contact numbers. Include medical ID cards current prescriptions.

Carry an extra set of batteries for the glucose meter (or insulin pump if a portable unit is used and requires them).

The glucagon emergency should include written, concise and easily understood instructions for its utilisation if not traveling with someone who knows how to administer it .

Set a travel alarm to ring 4 hourly as a reminder to continue regular eating habits when abroad and keep it by the pre packaged emergency snack.

Further Reading TravelPackeHow.co.uhttp://www.ehow.co.uk/how_6521103_prepare-diabetes-travel-pack.html#ixzz0vqcZIkEj

INFORMATION SOURCE Diabetes U.K. (formerly The British Diabetic Association)

George Kassianos . Iain B.McIntosh.

Chapter 8
Frail, disabled and handicapped travellers

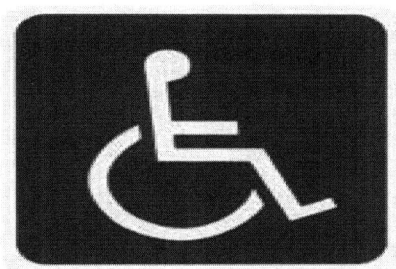

The physically frail, disabled and handicapped traveller

The majority of older travellers are relatively fit and aged between 65 and 80 years, with cruise ships often having a preponderance of senior passengers. Population trends indicate an increasing number of people living to 80 years and over. Many will have enjoyed previous global travel, or visits to relatives far afield and desire to venture abroad again. A considerable number of elderly travellers have some measure of physical incapacity. A minority will be physically disabled and be dependent upon walking aids and wheelchairs. Individual disabled travellers have successfully undertaken journeys to some of the world's most remote places. The determined, goal-orientated, physically challenged can and do make remarkable global voyages. In our society, holiday-making and travelling have become civic rights. Handicapped people however frequently find this "civic right to travel difficult to implement. Mobility barriers, unpleasant social-communicative contacts with non-disabled people and discrimination act as disincentives.[1]If they can overcome health and transportation hazards, international travel can widen restricted horizons and bring rich individual reward. Travel health professionals can facilitate the ease and comfort of the journey.

Some of the less able, intent on world travel suffer from loss of essential faculties and physical impairment due to stroke and chronic arthritis, or major joint surgery. Poor balance adds to mobility difficulties. Despite frailties most can travel where they will, with adequate preplanning and preparation. Some even find that transfer to a drier, sunny environment improves symptoms and enhances motility.

Physical handicap is not an insurmountable barrier to international journeying but, the need for cautious, anticipatory travel planning and medical assessment is a vital pre-requisite, if these travellers are to relocate in safety.

Pre-travel consultation. Most will benefit from pre travel health consultation. Proposed route, transportation mode and destination are major considerations in determining the additional hazards of travel presenting to handicapped. The health professional should be aware of the difficulties which can present to the disabled traveller especially if wheel chair bound. Gradually, access improvements are being made for travellers with disability who wish to holiday abroad. Ease of travel for these people revolves round the foreign location, local transport and accommodation facilities and the nature of the disability .The travel industry is slowly endeavouring to accommodate the needs of the less than physically perfect and their incapacity should not preclude desired international travel. However, increasing age is accompanied by increased incidence of stroke, Parkinson's disease, disabling arthritis, loss of function and faculties such as deafness and sight.

Inadequate, or non-existent, facilities for those physically disadvantaged are the norm in Third World and impoverished countries, and over much of Eastern Europe and Asia. Some societies are psychologically unprepared to recognise the special| needs of those functionally disabled and may even positively discriminate against those who are physically incapacitated. Sometimes, individuals suffering severe physical frailty, functional disability and handicap should be advised to restrict foreign travel to countries best equipped to accommodate their needs. Countries with the best facilities for the disabled are:-

United Kingdom and Ireland

Scandinavia

Northern Europe

Republic of South Africa

New Zealand

Australia

Hong Kong and Singapore

North America including the United States of America and Canada[2]

This does not mean that these countries present no problems for travellers, but there is state provision for those with functional incapacity. Psychologically too, the populations of these countries are likely to react positively in support of individuals with physical limitations. At local level in all countries, however, there may be failure to provide the support necessary to maintain the smooth progress of the physically challenged en route, or in transit. In some countries such as the United States of America antidiscrimination laws may inadvertently act to this groups disadvantage e.g. early flight boarding restrictions in some States.

Disabilities. Handicap and disability can be divided into categories such as visible and non-visible conditions, ambulatory and non-ambulatory with drop-foot, resulting from stroke, a visible, ambulatory condition and deafness a non-visible one. Public support is more likely to be offered for the former as the disability is obvious.

Pretravel documentation. The majority of travellers leave the UK. by air. People with acute and chronic conditions should complete and submit to the chosen airline in advance of the trip, the Medif form, as an indication that they are a passenger with special needs. The international air transport association has produced MEDIF and FREMEC cards for completion by disabled, potential passengers. Part 1 of the MEDIF, the 'INCAD' is a record of current incapacity to be completed by the passenger. Part 2 requires completion by the passenger's doctor. For most permanently disabled people, a medical report on current state is needed to permit airline transportation. The completion of a FREMEC form does not eliminate the need for prior notification of the disability for requirements of flight, but can be used to ease transit for frequent airline passengers. This data transfer is wholly dependent on accurate completion of questions by the patient and on patient willingness to complete the form in the first place. Many elderly patients and those who are physically incapacitated still present to airlines without having completed the forms and airline agents can refuse onward transportation. Prior notification of physical incapacity before a flight is essential to ensure appropriate support is available on the day of travel. Blind persons and people dependent upon walking aids and wheelchair transport will also have to advise transportation staff at train and bus stations and ports of their special needs in transit, boarding and disembarking

Deafness

Deafness is non-visible, strongly age-related and probably the most prevalent physical impairment in the old. About one-third of those over 75 years of age are affected to some degree and 20% over 80 years require hearing aids.[3] The older, deaf traveller runs the risk of missing important travel announcements at airports, rail and bus stations which may mean missed connections, but can be serious in the event of an emergency. Elderly travellers often switch off hearing aids when inundated by the cacophony of noise inseparable from busy transport transit points. Many people, whether they are hearing, deaf or have tinnitus, find that flying can cause pain or discomfort in ears, and temporary hearing loss

If travelling alone, the elderly very deaf person should inform the transport carrier and agencies of the need for special consideration. Couriers and travel stewards need to be briefed to keep a watchful eye upon them and ensure that there is adequate visual display information available. Many international airports now have special phone links for the hard of hearing, which use microcomputer technology. Deaf people can type in queries on a special telephone link and receive a typed reply in response.

Train travel for deaf and hearing impaired passengers has improved considerably with the introduction of new rolling stock and disability training for many front line staff.

When buying a ticket from the booking office at most major UK and European train stations it is usually possible to amplify sound via an induction loop system, with the switch set to the 'T' setting on the hearing aid. Most public address systems in airports should have induction loop facilities, Text phones and public telephones with amplification and induction loops should also be available. Staff at the airport information desk should be able to tell you where to find these.

Vision Support services for blind or visually impaired people at airports on request include someone to:

- meet and guide through check-in, baggage check and customs controls
- advise personally when plane is boarding if in a 'silent airport'
- help boarding of the plane and stow any luggage

At a security search, impairment should be explained to airport security staff and bags should be repacked in a specific order, so that essential items can be located.

Guide dogs should be allowed to travel free of charge, in the passenger cabin

Loss of visual acuity

Quarter of a million of the UK population is registered as blind or partially-sighted and 2 million have some sight loss with three quarters of the group over 65 years of age. [3] Nearly 90% of older people wear spectacles and studies suggest 20% of 80 year olds are unable to read newsprint even with prescribed spectacles. Cataract and age-related macular deterioration occur in 20 to 40% of persons between 65-74 years with glaucoma affecting 20 % of others.[4]

Hypertropia-(far sightedness) where the point of focus lies behind the retina is the most common refractive defect,

Myopia (near sightedness) occurs where the point of focus is in front of the retina.

Presbyopia -an error in the refractive abilities of the eye - is a hypertropia for near vision. It develops with advancing age and results from a physiological change in the accommodative mechanisms by which the focus of the eye is adjusted for objects seen at different distances. The lens gradually becomes less pliable and eventually cannot accommodate in response to the action of the lens muscles. With a resultant failure to focus well for near vision .Remedial action is possible by wear of corrective spectacles.

Cataract may be caused by senile degeneration, with gradual, painless loss of vision. If the opacity is in the centre of the lens short sightedness develops early and a presbyopic person may discover that they can read without glasses .The condition is treatable with corrective spectacles and surgery, with cataract surgery most frequently performed surgical operation in western society.

Senile macular degeneration is a leading cause of visual impairment in the elderly and there is no known predisposing factor.

Many older people now spend long vacations, in countries with near constant high intensity day time sunlight. These two factors may see a rise in cataract formation and macular degeneration. One cause of cataract is oxidation which can be due to light damage and there are reports of increased cataract incidence in parts of the world exposed to strong sunlight for long periods.[5]

Light radiation reaching the eye passes to the retina and the macular part of it in particular, where it is absorbed by photoreceptors, usually protected from the harmful effects of light wavelengths in the ultraviolet range of visible light. With age the efficacy of the protection declines. Wearing good quality sunglasses is recommended for older people who venture into strong sunlight particularly when abroad. 'Wrap-around glasses offer best protection.

Logistically the disability accounts for fewer travel problems than might be expected. Blind people are not welcome on sea voyages because of inherent shipboard dangers, but cannot be excluded from shipping. In many countries guide dogs cannot accompany blind passengers on external flights across borders, without the dog undergoing lengthy quarantine. In countries such as UK and USA, "Seeing Eye" dogs are permitted to ride in the cabin of the aircraft with the disabled owner.

Blind passengers using canes are usually allowed to retain them by their seat on aircraft, but stringent application of security regulations sometimes means that canes are taken away by over-zealous authorities. Swiss airports regard walking poles as offensive weapons and will not permit them into the cabin of the aircraft.[6] Stewardesses will normally provide information regarding seat row position and guide a blind passenger to appropriate seating and toilet facilities. Airlines exclude blind persons from sitting in exit row seats to ensure the safety of aircraft and passengers. Some discriminatory airline practices are alleged to refuse to allow blind persons to sit at emergency exits, requiring them to sit in rear of the plane, requiring persons with dog guides to sit in bulkhead seats, requiring blind persons to pre-board, or be sequestered in a special holding area prior to boarding, or be subjected to special safety briefings and emergency instructions to wait until other passengers have deplaned before attempting exit. Many of these seem sensible safeguards to benefit all passengers.

Ensuring safe travel in elderly, blind and partly sighted people may require travel with a sighted companion. For educational and other purposes, blind passengers can travel with an escort at reduced rates on British internal flights. Sound health in the travel companion is important.

Case History.*The companion to a blind person fell on the first day of a rough weather cruise breaking the left arm and right clavicle .She found it impracticable to guide the blind person around and he was confined to the cabin for the remainder of the cruise.*

The introduction of modern rolling stock, better station facilities and staff training has improved the experience of travel by train for disabled passengers but it is important give advance warning to the railway company before the journey to allow support to be put in place. Modern rolling stock often has automated announcements advising station approach. A member of staff should assist train ascent and descent. On many trains, there are Braille buttons for opening doors as well as toilet doors.[7] The train will also have external doors that contrast with the body and interior hand rails of a contrasting colour, to help visually impaired passengers.

Major stations, such as those in cities, will have audio announcements, as well as visual screens, informing passengers of arrivals, departures, platform numbers and any delays that may occur. Most platforms now have a tactile edge near the running line to let blind and visually impaired passengers know that they are close to the railway line. Unfortunately these refinements which ease travel for the impaired will not be available in train travel across many other parts of the world.

Physical and locomotor disability

There are approximately 10 million adults in Britain who suffer from some form of disability and the Leonard Cheshire Charity which supports disabled people warns that airports still fail to meet their needs, despite EU laws introduced in 2008 that make it the responsibility of the airports to provide special assistance. Travel companies are also failing in this respect. "Tourism for all", another charity organisation, found that 80% of disabled respondents believed that travel agents failed to appreciate their needs and 35% would not consider booking with a main stream agent for this reason. Expedia the online travel firm has launched new search tools to aid disabled travellers find accessible accommodation.

Arthritis and hip replacement may restrict access to trains, aeroplanes and coaches, and the confined space of long-haul flights may create severe cramps and spasm in fixed limbs.[8] Loss of joint mobility may result in difficulty in accommodating limbs to the narrow confines of the aircraft cabin. Cramped legs may increase the risk of development of deep vein thrombosis. Poor balance and postural instability, a feature of ageing, adds to the risk of falls which are a common occurrence in older passengers in the unstable environment on cruise ships [9]Passengers should be advised to pre-book aircraft, coach and train seating, practicable some weeks before departure, to take advantage of seat positions with additional leg space. They should avoid seating next to the body of an aircraft, facing bulkheads and where it is impossible to recline seats. The obvious seat positions where there is extra space, at emergency exits, are denied to the elderly and the incapacitated as airline regulations stipulate that only the fit can occupy this seating, only allocated 24 hours before travel. However, an aisle seat has much to commend it for elderly travellers, as this allows extension of at least one limb into the passageway and eases exit from seating for exercise and toilet purposes. Assistance for passengers with special needs is now the responsibility of a Passenger with Reduced Mobility (PRM) team, employed by the airport and paid for by airlines. A PRM agent is responsible for boarding and seating disabled passengers.

Ships without lifts can prove an insurmountable hazard for those with fixed knees and hip deformities. Stairs and companionways can be narrow and steep on board ship, and seven to ten deck levels are commonplace. Transit of these areas in a swaying vessel is likely to cause falls in elderly people. Those with spastic limbs from stroke disease may also find similar restrictions to those suffered by the arthritic when travelling by sea or air.

Management

- Purchase of 'executive' or 'club class' tickets to win extra leg room if affluent.
- Buying entry to executive lounges where feet can be elevated and exercise taken before and between flights and until a late call to emplane.
- Exercise limbs and avoid venous stasis and possible pulmonary embolism in restricted seating on a protracted airline or coach journey.
- Use of constrictive pressure stockings on protracted trips
- Use of a walking pole for additional support.

Locomotion difficulties from imbalance and disabled limbs create difficulties on stairs, long walkways, on lurching companionways and decks, with a real risk of falls and fracture in older passengers. Passengers should consider the facilities, lift availability and the suitability of a cruise ship for their particular needs as carefully as choice of cabin. Older ships have fewer lifts, limited disabled occupancy cabins and steep stairs, but newer ships have wide passages and stairways and many open spaces with a dearth of handrails. Access to life boats and emergency disembarkation should also be considered as lifts are rendered inoperative in the event of fire, or flooding. 10

Incontinence problems.

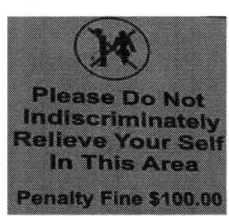

Toilet access and continence are topics rarely considered by travel agents, but exercise the mind of many intending older travellers. The question of toilet access en route and on holiday is a prominent travel related anxiety. 11UK or foreign travel brings inevitable restrictions on toilet access and variable toilet facilities. Abroad these are often coupled with limited water supply, inadequate sanitation and poor hygiene. This prospect can be daunting for those with good bladder control.It can inhibit the will to travel in those with urinary problems, fearful of possible loss of bladder control and urinary embarrassment, while in the public domain. Senescence per se does not cause incontinence, although ageing can affect the lower urinary tract and predispose to it. Some degree of occasional or regular incontinence is common among elderly people with up to 71% of those living in the community being affected. Estimates suggest that there are 1 million sufferers within the UK, the majority being citizens over the age of 65 and most being women.[11] Many are too embarrassed to discuss their functional disturbance and surveys have shown that only 1 in 5 is prepared to discuss this problem with a health professional. The affliction causes many to avoid far travel from home. The mildly affected, sometimes pressurised into travel by spouse or offspring, may allow their fears to surface at pre-travel interview. The cause, in absence of a surgical disturbance, is usually due to bladder instability resulting from an uninhibited neurogenic bladder, which gives rise to urge incontinence, or sphincter weakness giving stress incontinence. Several management procedures can relieve symptoms, bring control, or make the condition sufficiently manageable for the individual to travel without undue concern[12].These should be instituted in the months prior to travel.

Those with normal bladder function, but with other physical disabilities may also meet with functional toilet difficulties while travelling in foreign countries. Poor locomotion or transport abilities, imbalance and lower joint stiffness, or rigidity are likely to create problems in toilets commonly met in transcontinental travel. Toilets traditional to the host country may cater for only those who can squat unaided over a plumbing fixture no more than a tiled hole in the ground.

In continental Europe and the UK. where sanitary units may be more conventional, toilet seats may also be absent. The ability to hover over a toilet bowl, or perch upon porcelain, in the absence of toilet rails and wall supports, is a skill often beyond the ability of the old, with arthritic joints and poor spinal function.

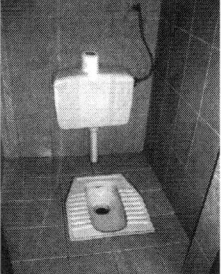

Even if older women can manage this functional procedure, there is a 21% reduction in normal urine flow rate and 19% increase in residual urine volume in the crouching position forcing further toileting shortly.[13] This, associated with poor renal clearance and the possibility of dehydration and infection on a visit to a tropical country, may lead to serious urinary tract problems sufficient to ruin the vacation. At best, the women with urinary anxieties on a coach tour will be inhibited by the queue to reach the toilet and the line of women waiting impatiently for entry while she micturates.

In aircraft, trains, ships and coaches accessing toilet accommodation in a lurching, swaying conveyance can risk loss of balance and a fall. Grab handles may be at a premium in the convenience, seating may be too low for the less agile and floors can be awash making bladder relief a dreaded experience. Aircraft cabin staff can assist passengers to the toilet, but food handler status pre-empts them from providing assistance in the toilet, a consideration some disabled passengers fail to appreciate. The peripheral siting of rest rooms in stations and airports can also defeat elderly people faced with a long walk to find relief. Inadequately signposted loos are another traveller's hazard and communication difficulties can add to the trauma of the search. The difference between senora and senore is none too obvious to the linguistically challenged.

Public toilets are rare in developing countries and when available are frequently poorly maintained and unhygienic. Toilet paper and hand-washing facilities are luxuries denied to much of the world's populace. Free toilet access is rare and toilet guardians will deny access no matter how great the need for entry, in the absence of appropriate coinage of the country. Coaches in Eastern Europe and developing countries are likely to be without facilities and cramped for space. Onerous demands placed on the bowel by gastroenteritis, the scourge of travellers, with diarrhoea and frequent defecation needs, can further add to individual discomfiture when voiding facilities are inadequate.

Advised of the paucity and variation in toilet facilities common to foreign travel, the elderly traveller can usually, with sensible preparation, overcome many of these sanitary deficiencies. The informed doctor advising older patients on healthy travel can also help minimise problems relating to feared or actual incontinence.

The disorder is frequently neglected, poorly evaluated and ineffectively treated by family doctors. Improved bladder control can enhance the quality of life and can encourage travel. Fundamentally, the condition is due to over or under activity of detrusor function, or sphincter dysfunction, involving internal or external sphincter, or a combination of both. Infections, medications, loss of muscle tone, and diabetes are other relevant features in elderly women.

Males suffer less from incontinence but they too can have urinary problems which can spoil a foreign holiday. Urgency from prostatism demands immediate access to a toilet often denied by the waiting queue in long haul aircraft. Difficulties are likely to relate to prostatic hypertrophy and acute retention. Exposure to cheap wines and spirits often found abroad and on aircraft can lead to excessive alcohol ingestion and acute retention, if the prostate is enlarged. Prolonged intervals between bladder voiding due to transit delays and lack of toilet access can precipitate inability to urinate. This may only result in painful embarrassment and the inconvenience of a trip to a casualty unit if the journey involves a UK coach tour, but abroad it may have more serious consequences.

Case history

A fit, retired 67 year old school teacher on a coach tour to Devon from Scotland suffered an acute retention when his much-delayed coach, devoid of a toilet, was held up in a traffic jam on the motorway. He was admitted to an emergency unit,was catheterised and advised to have a trans-urethral resection. This was done shortly after admission, the operation was successful and he was fit enough to catch his coach on its return journey north. Another 72 year old was less fortunate. He had always wanted to view the Himalayas and on this holiday of a life-time he finally reached Kathmandu. Unable to resist the call of the mountains, he arranged a few days trekking in the Himalayan foothills. The second night out from base, he suffered an acute retention. A passing medic in another trekking group was asked to help. In the absence of a catheter, the retention was relieved by the passage of a stethoscope tube. Although this brought immediate relief, he developed a urinary infection, became pyrexial, then dehydrated. He had to be evacuated back to the capital and, in the absence of wheeled transport, was carried out of the high valleys on the back of a Sherpa porter. Even in hospital his convalescence was protracted and he was very relieved to ultimately return to NHS care and subsequent operation.

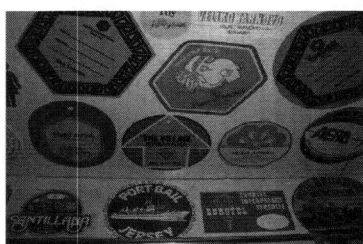
Travel Plans

Management

The pre-travel consultation allows nurse or doctor to tactfully explore with the patient any apprehensions regarding continence. If none are admitted the opportunity should be taken to advise on the variability of access and the quality of toilet facilities likely to be met in international airports and different countries, stressing the inadequacy of those in the third world.

An information hand-out can reinforce instructions. Acquisition of passenger leaflets from British Airport Authority airports, detailing toilet access, should be advised.

Elderly American ladies, on the 'Blue Rinse' route through the States, travel with a clutch of paper toilet seat covers, a precaution more appropriate to antiquated washroom fittings in Europe than in the USA and a safeguard which could be appropriate for other elderly travellers abroad. One old lady patient, an intrepid traveller to far-away places and very familiar with the uncrowned toilet bowls of foreign parts, actually carries her own light-weight, plastic toilet-seat cover with her on her travels!

Ensconced within the tight confines of an aircraft or coach toilet, the old are likely to come to little harm, but traversing aisles and passages in ships on choppy seas or in lurching planes, trains or buses, they run the risk of falls and fractures. Use of a folding walking pole should be suggested, for accessing toilet accommodation on moving transport.

Given enough time before travel, those with occasional incontinence, or regular disturbance, can often be helped to overcome the problem, or make it manageable during travel. Patients may have to be coaxed into giving details of frequency, urgency, nocturia, dribbling and involuntary voiding with coughing and sneezing. These features help identify urgency and dribbling incontinence and provide pointers to management[14,15] The nurse can obtain the history with the use of simple questionnaires on bladder control .The doctor should make a physical examination of pelvis, rectum and vagina to identify any specific causative factor and referred to the appropriate specialist consultant.

 Most patients will be female and urinary tract infections, atrophic vaginitis, cystocoele and rectal overloading have to be considered and treated if found. Prostatism requires a rectal check and PSA investigation. Review of diuretics, hypnotics and sedatives is required. An MSU should be checked for infection and glycosuria. Patients should be encouraged to keep diary records of toilet demands and frequency, urinary volumes and number of incontinence pads used.

All too often no specific correctable cause will be found, but bladder retraining exercises and drug therapy can still help many of these potential travellers.

Causes of urinary incontinence

1   Detrusor instability - when the bladder muscle or detrusor contracts uninhibitedly - giving rise to urge incontinence, frequency, enuresis and stress incontinence.

2 Urethral sphincter incompetence–where urethral resistance is decreased and stress incontinence occurs.

3 Both conditions can coexist. Both frequently respond to treatment which needs to be instituted at least three months before departure on holiday

Treatment

If detrusor instability is not due to a neuropathy, bladder retraining is recommended. Retraining instruction involves emphasis on voiding at certain times and holding on for as long as possible. Stress incontinence can respond to pelvic floor exercises which young elderly individuals can tackle and practise with success.

The traveller who suffers episodic symptoms of instability with stressful events e.g airport transit, aircraft take off, can be given a musculotrophic drug such as oxybutynin as it had a short half-life, Drug treatment of overflow incontinence is not very successful.

If there is little benefit from drugs, exercises and retraining, the provision of adequate incontinence aids such as Kanga pants and incontinence pads may make short and medium distance travel a practicality for those determined on global travel. Urisheaths, catheters and leg bags can be managed successfully en route by older patients, as long as intellectual impairment does not impair good control.

History

History taking by nurse or doctor should include:

Questions on:	destination and transportation
	have you any worries about toilet access on the journey?
	do you have to get up at night ?
	do you sometimes not make it to the toilet?
	do you leak urine when you exercise, sneeze, run, cough,?
	do you have problems actually emptying the bladder?
Investigations	Mid stream specimen of urine (organisms, sugar albumen)
	Prostatic specific antibody test

Advice: Possibility of - limited facilitie - no wash-hand basins, toilet paper, toilet seats, toilet bowls, wall supports, grab handles, privacy

Non-availability on airside of customs and immigration, during protracted holding manoeuvres before aircraft landing/take off, and in developing countries

Preparation: hand luggage carriage of toilet paper, toilet seat covers, incontinence aids, appropriate continence-inducing drugs

Examination by doctor (if incontinence admitted)

Vaginal and rectal examination to exclude infection, atrophy, cystocoele, rectal over-loading and prostatism

Prescription Prescribe oxybutinin twice daily as a trial, at least 3 weeks before departure, or if the problem is anxiety-related, to be taken before the stressful event

Stress incontinence: -Instruction in pelvic floor exercises with the patient taught to practise interrupted micturition every time she goes to the toilet and to carry out the exercises 8-!" times per day. A large number of sufferers can be cured if they carry out this regime.

Urge incontinence - secondary to bladder instability

Bladder drill and retraining is highly successful in compliant patients. Patients are allowed only to go to the toilet at certain times, which are progressively lengthened every two days.

Wheelchair Traveller.

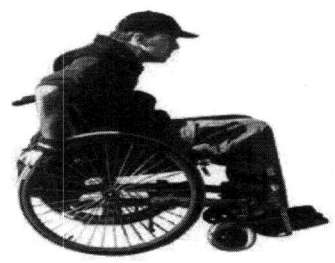

Wheel chair travellers face access problems with most transport and accommodation in over-seas travel.[xvi] They must consider aircraft size, ramp access wheel chair carriage and transit stopovers. The latter should be a major consideration as transit points on long haul flights may utilise an airport in the Middle East or the Gulf states with few aids for the disabled traveller. It is vital that at no point in long haul travel with transfers that a small plane is used on a feeder service. Most large international airports now have adequate rampage and wheelchair access and this is true of the majority of cruise ships. Coaches and trains however, even on conventional tours and routes have variable ease of access. Trains stations often mean dependency upon lifts which may or may not be operative. Between-deck lifts on ships may not be available in rough weather, or emergency situations, such as fire. British law (since 1996) makes it an offence for providers of goods and services to provide inferior service to a disabled person because of their disability. The Act on Accessibility (1999) to transport, applies only to new trains from 1999 and coaches from 2000.and does not apply to air and sea travel.

Careful, early pre-planning and organisation will smooth the way to safe journey.Competition between travel services ensures variability and medical counsellors should be prepared to discuss the benefits of ''shopping around' in ensuring that passage is with a caring carrier.

Air travel

Prior to purchase of a flight ticket the wheelchair bound should complete the appropriate forms requested by airline management -Incapacitated Passengers Handling Advice (INCAD) form and/or a Medical Information Form (MEDIF (see chap.7) In smaller airports, wheelchair access and provision may be inadequate or non-existent xvi At these locations disabled passengers may have to be manually lifted from the aircraft down steps by airport employees. Large airliners now carry skychairs - on board wheelchairs which expedite movement to the toilet.

Personal transportation of a lightweight wheelchair is advised even when passengers are accustomed to a battery operated one, as they are easy to store on board. Electric chairs are unwieldy heavy vehicles and carriage of batteries is often restricted by airlines. The carrying of electric wheelchairs is allowed. An electric wheelchair will be classed as a dangerous material on account of its battery being considered a hazard. A wheelchair powered by a battery that could spill must have the batteries entirely removed. Batteries that cannot spill, do not have to be removed from the chair .Airlines must carry mobility equipment free of charge but many airlines only allow one wheelchair per plane.

The physically handicapped may have to consider travelling with a companion to expedite transit changeovers and provide en route support. Some airlines, charge a nominal fee only for the carriage of such a travel supporter. To travel alone the passenger should be capable of moving from a passenger seat to an on board wheelchair, as cabin crew are prohibited from lifting passengers in and out of seats.

For safety reasons, airlines are entitled to require that the disabled person travels with a companion if not 'self-reliant.

To travel by air alone, the traveller must be capable of:
•unfastening seat belt
•leaving seat and reaching an emergency exit unaided
•donning an oxygen mask and lifejacket
•understanding safety briefing and instructions, given by the crew in emergency.

If help is required for feeding, medication or toilet, a travel companion is needed

Every airport in the UK now offers free assistance for disabled passengers to reach and leave planes. The Passenger with reduced mobility (PRM) team is responsible for boarding and seating disabled passengers. This applies to visible and non-visible disability.

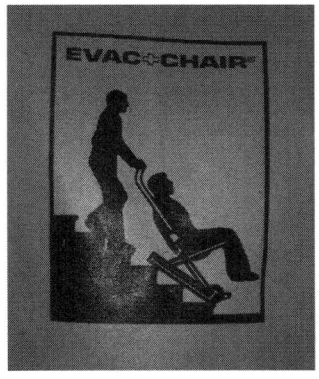

Recommended Airlines

Air Canada - This airline provides good support within the airport and assistance on board, with regularly checks to ensure all is well. On most flights, extra seating is available at no extra cost if needed due to disability. Service animals are allowed provided they can sit at the feet without protruding into the aisle.

Continental Airlines - The airline offers special seating arrangements and on board assistance, including help for those with mobility problems whether or not they use wheelchairs. They welcome service animals and have a special onboard kennel to make them more comfortable.

EasyJet - EasyJet will arrange assistance to get to plane-side with a lift up any steps in a carry chair if necessary. Some support is available onboard but there are no aisle wheelchairs. Safety instructions are provided separately for visually impaired and hearing impaired passengers. Service animals can only travel on domestic flights.

Quantas Quantas, provides full support from the moment of arrival at the airport, will lift passenger in and out of seat if needed, and arranges early boarding. Service animals are welcome and, if a carer is needed both customer and carer travel at reduced rate.

Virgin Atlantic - This airline provides a good support service for visually impaired and hearing impaired passengers and passengers with mental disabilities who choose to travel alone. There's limited support for mobility impaired people, with spacious adapted toilets on longer flights. Service animals are welcome to travel in the cabin on most major routes.

Airlines must carry mobility equipment free of charge. Disabled travellers must advise the airline when booking the flight with details of wheelchair or scooter, particularly if a powered wheelchair or scooter. Seating on board an aircraft has to meet air safety regulations. The wheelchair will be stored in the hold of the plane.It is usually possible for the passenger to stay in their wheelchair until plane-side before transfer to an on-board chair, an easy task if there is an air bridge connection..If the plane is parked away from the terminal, passengers will to use a flight of stairs to board, or a scissor lift, If the wheelchair has to be specially packed, it may be necessary to transfer into an airport chair at check-in, especially if a powered wheelchair or scooter.

Under European law, disabled people and other people with reduced mobility have legal rights to assistance when travelling by air. Airlines are not obliged to fly disabled passengers who are flown at their discretion. There are only two specific reasons why they may deny flying access. The first is if there may be a danger to other passengers. The second consideration is the risk of requirement for urgent medical attention which could force flight diversion.

Medications

A chronically ill and infirm person is allowed to take all medicines needed onto the flight, even if that means exceeding the usual security allowance for liquids. These should be in their original containers with liquids packed separately in a clear plastic bag. Extra water can be carried if needed for health reasons. Prescription liquid medications and other liquids needed by persons with disabilities and medical conditions include:

All prescription and over-the-counter medications (liquids, gels, and aerosols) including petroleum jelly, eye drops, and saline solution for medical purposes;

Liquids including water, juice, or liquid nutrition or gels Life-support and life-sustaining liquids such as bone marrow, blood products, Frozen items are allowed as long as they are frozen solid when presented for screening. If the liquid medications are in volumes larger than 3.4 ounces (100ml) each, they may not be placed in the quart-size bag and must be declared to the Transportation Security Officer. A declaration of content can be made verbally, in writing, or by a person's companion, caregiver, interpreter, or family member.

Declared liquid medications and other liquids for disabilities and medical conditions must be kept separate from all other property submitted for x-ray screening. Repeat prescription forms for the medication should be carried with a list of medications and preferably a note as to their need signed by the family doctor

Coach Travel

Pre-enquiry must include availability of a mechanical wheelchair lift, or employees willing to manually assist passenger and whether the wheelchair can be secured to the floor, the passage permits transfer from wheelchair to seat and there is access to on board toilet? Novice travellers must be aware that in many parts of the developing world tourist coaches will have no toilet and be cramped for space. Local buses if available, will be grossly overloaded, with a scramble for seats at each stop.

Train Travel

There may not only be a gap between platform and carriage but many continental trains have carriage doors raised high above ground. Porterage is now rare at many stations. On board toilets can be squalid, unhygienic and with flooded floors. Assistance may be only a bell press away, but speedy aid is dependent on the cooperation of a conductor often many coaches away

Cruise ship travel

Many of the large ships have excellent disabled passenger cabins and adequacy of between deck lifts but older ships still suffer from passage, toilet access and stair obstructions. Transfer to shore by ship's tender is still common with ladders to be negotiated on and off the ship. Gang planks can be steep and even in benign weather, negotiating broad ship spaces can be challenging. In rough weather wheelchairs can be tilted over.

Despite many advances in access to airports and stations aircraft, trains and coaches in the developed world, travelling with a wheelchair remains a challenge and transport services are not user friendly. In the developing world and many foreign parts the experience can prove daunting with vagaries that the best of planning cannot anticipate. Safe world travel is however feasible for most elderly disabled people guided to realistic goals, on carefully pre-planned individualised journeys. Travelling with a supporter alleviates many problems in transit but their personal health is also a consideration.

Case History. A severely disabled lady accompanied by her spouse was travelling to the Arctic on a cruise ship accommodated in a disabled person's cabin. She required assistance feeding toileting and getting to bed. Halfway to Greenland the husband had a severe heart attack and had to be helicoptered to the distant mainland. The wife was left bereft of care. Medical and nursing staff coping with a norovirus outbreak could not help, nor were cruise staff permitted by regulation to give intimate support. Goodwill and ad hoc temporary arrangements provided basic feeding and toilet assistance until she too was flown out on a casualty evacuation flight to Norway in a very expensive repatriation exercise.

Charities supporting disabled people report that leading travel companies are failing to serve the needs of disabled travellers. 85% of disabled respondents did not believe that travel agents understood their needs or catered for them. [17]Accommodation and access problems regularly arose with bookings and the traveller needs to confirm that these considerations have been addressed before travel.

Elevator and Facilities Access

A lift size 3ft.10 in. deep, 2ft.6in. wide is necessary for wheelchairs with a maximum of 2 steps for negotiation. Lavatories must have dimensions of 5ft. 4in x 3ft.7in. to allow man internal wheelchair manoeuvre. Entrance doors should be at least 2ft. 6in. wide and walkways ramped where necessary.[18]

Summary

- World travel is feasible for elderly disabled people on customised journeys.
- Counsellors must guide towards realistic goals and anticipate problems
- They should consider travel with healthy spouse, or independent, supporter.
- They should be directed towards support organisations for further advice on travel arrangements.
- Safe travel in the frail elderly and handicapped passenger demands careful pretravel planning, competent medical assessment, sound counselling and a user friendly transport mode and destination.

Within acceptable parameters, world travel need not be out of reach for those with physical and functional limitations. It can expand restricted horizons and be a worthwhile venture.

DISABLED TRAVELLER INSTRUCTION LEAFLET
Ten Tips for Healthy Travel

The ease of travel for a person with a disability depends upon destination, transport and accommodation facilities, .Plan and prepare in advance before travel abroad.

Plan ahead,

1 **Discuss with travel agent** accessibility of transport and accommodation, especially if using a wheelchair. If you require assistance for a flight you will be required to complete an 'Incapacitated PassengersHandling Advice' (INCAD) form. The second part of this form 'Medical   Information Form' (MEDIF) needs to be filled in by your Doctor if you have a medical condition.

2.**Seek advice early** for immunisations, malaria prevention, health education, fitness to fly certificate, medical facilities in destination country.

3 **Be honest in stating degree of disability.**

4 **Acquire medical insurance cover**, making sure emergency repatriation is included and maintenance or replacement costs for physical aids, mobility or medical equipment are included.

5 **Prepare for the journey**: How do you plan to get to the airport, access transport, store of aids or equipment, obtain assistance, order special diets ,access toilet facilities on aeroplane, train or boat?

6 **Carry any medication** required in hand luggage for journey and destination. Carry prescription repeat forms and list of medications and doctors letter for injections. Wear a medicalert bracelet if appropriate.

7 **Maintain hydration.** Before departure by plane, boat or train, do not reduce fluid intake to reduce the need to go to the toilet. It is important, particularly for flying, that you maintain fluid intake.

8 **Do leg exercises** during journeys when sitting a long time.

9 **Confirm destination arrangements.** How will you be met and who will meet you at the airport if you need assistance.

10 **Carry names of contacts** and telephone numbers of contacts at destination should plans go astray.

11.**Carry a language phrase book** and learn key assistance phrases before departure.

CHECK LIST FOR TRAVELLERS WITH EXISTING HEALTH PROBLEMS[18]

- Arrange a full medical check up several weeks before departure
- Ensure adequate and inclusive medical insurance cover including repatriation.
- Consider whether the special form should be completed to advise transport agents of disability before departure by air
- Advise airlines of special medical, dietary and mobility requirements
- Re-assess medication before departure. Drug review should pay special attention to diuretics, insulin, hypnotics, H2 antagonists, anticholinergics, anti epileptics and interactions with anti-malarials.
- Adequate medication should be carried in the hand luggage.
- Be aware of special risks of high altitude and, climate extremes.
- consider the need for supplemental oxygen.if potential respiratory problems in aircraft
- Consider adjustment of food intake and insulin dosage if diabetic
- On long haul flights endeavour to exercise legs as often as possible and avoid staying immobile for long periods
- Be aware that medical ,transport and toilet facilities en route and at destination may be of poor standard.
- Disabled cruise passengers should check the adequacy of medical and access facilities before booking

Useful Contacts :

The Disabled Living Foundation - information on flying and travel advice. 380-384 Harrow Road, London W9 2HU Tel 0171 289 6111

The Royal Institute for the Blind -information on tape for flying and travelling. 224 Great Portland Street, London W1N 6AA. Tel : 0171 388 1266

Royal Association for Disability and Rehabilitation (RADAR) produce information for disability and travel.12 City Forum, 250 City Road, London EC1V 8AF. Tel : 0171 250 3222

Heathrow Airport -Free guide to facilities 'Traveller's Information Special Needs. Tel 0181 745 7495

Extensive Advice on Travel for the Disabled at Disabled Travel . www.disabledtraveladvice.co.uk

Resources.

Health Advice for Travellers. Department of Health -. Available free from post offices. Contains basic travel health advice, recommended immunisations, information about travel insurance and entitlement to medical treatment in the European Community

www.direct.gov.uk/DisabledPeople/TravelHolidaysAndBreaks

LaGrow S, Wiener W, LaDuke R. Independent travel for developmentally disabled persons: a comprehensive model of instruction Res Dev Disabil. 1990 ;11(3):289-301.

wwwjid.sagepub.com/content/2/4/195.refs

Airline access ruleswww.allgohere.com

Further reading

- "Nothing Ventured: Disabled People Travel the World". Walsh A (1991) (Lonely Planet Series), Harrup Columbus, (ISBN 0747 102082).
- Travel and Health in the Elderly A Medical Handbook. McIntosh I, 1992. Quay Books, Mark Allan Publications, London.
- Health Hazard and the high risk traveller. McIntosh I, 1993. Quay Books, Mark Allan Publications, London.
- Travellers Health. Fourth Edition, Ed. Dawood R. Oxford University Press, Oxford 2002

Travel medicine and Migrant Health Ed Lockie C Walker E et al 2000 Churchill :Livingstone . Edinburgh.Chap. 7 McIntosh I

National Suppliers of Medical Goods

Travel Medical Centre Ltd. Provide Sterile Injection. Kits (with Intra-fusion drips)Charlotte Keel Health Centre
Seymour Rd Eastern Bristol BS5 0UA

Homeway Promotions Ltd Provide Range of Travel Goods

The White House .Littleton Winchester .Hampshire. SO22
Industrial Pharmaceutical Service Ltd. Provide Travel Sterile Packs only. Bridgewater Rd.Broadheath
Altrincham Cheshire WA14 1NA
Philip Harris Medical Ltd. Provide Travel Aid Kit with sterile syringes, dioralyte
SafariQuip   AccessibleGuide.co.uk/FreeGuide

References

1 Mitchell M Have wheelchair will travel. 1995. Travel Medicine Internat. 13(5)174.7
2 McIntosh I 1995 travel and Health in the Elderly. Quay Books . Mark Allan Pub. Dinton Somerset
3 Keyinformationandstatisticshttp://www.rnib.org.uk/aboutus/Research/statistics/Pages/statistics.aspx
4 http://www.rnib.org.uk/aboutus/Research/statistics/Pages/statistics.aspx
5 Neale RE, Purdie JL, Hirst LW, Green AC Neale RE, Purdie JL, Hirst LW, Green AC Sun exposure as a risk factor for nuclear cataract Epidemiology. 2003 Nov;14(6):707-12..
6 In the News British Trav. Health Assoc. J 2010.2
7 Dessary BL. Robin MR. Fasini W. (1997) The aged infirm or handicapped traveller in Textbook of travel medicine and health. Ed. Steffen R. DuPont HL. Decker Pub. Canada
8Dargent-Molina P, Favier F, et al (1996). Poorer balance and postural stability make falls more likely. Lancet, 348; 145-9.
9 McIntosh I Power K Reed J Prevalence and intensity of travel related stressors.1996 J Trav. Med.96-102
10Mandelstam D (1986). Incontinence and its Management 2 edn. Croon Helm, London McIntosh I. Health and safety at sea. 1997 Trav. Med. Inter.15.234-7
11Brocklehurst JC Urinary incontinence in the community--analysis of a MORI poll. BMJ. 1993 Mar 27;306 (6881):832-4.
12 O'Dowd T, MD, FRCGP, Management of urinary incontinence in women British Journal of General Practice, 1993, 43, 426-429.
13 Moore K, Richmond D et al (1991). Crouching Over the Toilet, Brit J Obs Gyn, 98, 569-72
14 Jolleys J (1988). Diagnosis and Management of Urinary Incontinence in Females in General Practice, BMJ, 296,1300-02
15 Fanti J et al (1991). Efficacy of Bladder Retraining in Older Women with Incontinence, JAmerMed
16 Stewart M Physical impairment and global travel Brit. J. travel health 2010.14
17McIntosh I Disabled travel. In the news. Brit. J. travel health 2010. 15.58
18 McIntosh I. Advice for disabled travellers. In the news Brit. J. travel health 200811.54

Iain B. McIntosh

Chapter 9

Psychological aspects of global travel and older people.

Global travel is part of life style for many older people. A sizeable proportion of the population however, both old and young, are fearful of travelling by air, under and over water, a prerequisite for those departing from Britain. The phobic may exhibit avoidance behaviour and refuse to contemplate leaving the UK.to the disadvantage of spouse and partner. Recent climatic, terrorist and financial events have made all forms of transportation a more worrying experience adding to common fears of travel in a ship, aircraft, or through a long tunnel.

Realistic concerns about aeroplane mechanical failure do not now predominate as in early days of aircraft travel, but recent well publicised events have enhanced worries about this mode of transportation. The financial recession has resulted in airline economies bringing decline in customer care and failure to address passenger's legitimate anxieties regarding airport congestion, luggage loss, flight delays, cancellations and rerouting.

Air travel is regarded as the most dangerous and anxiety provoking travel option by the general public. 1 Flight anxiety is an emotional state of worry triggered by an appreciation of risks usually disproportionate to the actual risks involved in air travel. Recent media reports of thousands of travellers marooned for days in airports in Britain and Europe has altered public perception of risk relating to air transportation and focused it on airports.

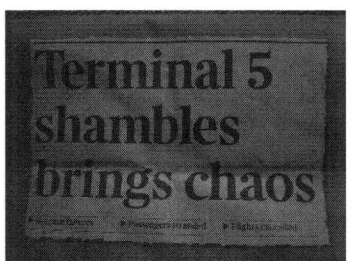

Phenomenal loss of luggage, cancelled flights, rerouting and stranding has however brought anxieties about this travel mode more in line with the proportionate risk of an unwanted event occurring to the traveller. Paradoxically as the risk of mechanical aeroplane failure and physical danger has waned the likelihood of major psychological trauma in air travel has increased markedly. Major delays, prolonged waits in packed airline lounges, vast queues in airports and the uncertainty of arrival and departure have impacted on the public psyche. Land and sea transport has not been exempted from weather and terrorist anomalies, with passengers marooned on motorways and rail lines and in terminals.

These events are bringing behavioural change, particularly in seniors. The old are more psychologically vulnerable to uncontrolled situations .Common features of old age such as indecisiveness, slower problem solving, inflexibility in purpose, poorer memory and cognitive decline aggravate personal reaction to the frenzied environment in airports and rail stations, when all onward movement abruptly ceases. Pre-flight worries and anxieties are added to the concerns older travellers have of actually flying. Their cumulative effect can promote tension and angst with the psychological effects resulting in adverse physiological responses, cardiac stress and possible heart attack and stroke.

There was a fall in air travel in 2010 disproportionate to that relating to financial recession. Saga travel, an operator specialising in elderly travel, reported a coinciding increase in passengers seeking to avoid the fly part of the cruise experience by use of UK ports for arrival and departure. The Passenger Shipping Association stated that 650,000 passengers shunned airports and set sail from a UK port in 2010, 10% more than in the previous year. Older people who are not time-pressurised like the young, are avoiding potentially stress-provoking airports.

Older people also often have a wealth of travel experience of adverse events relating to air travel which may generate fears and anxieties, not affecting the phlegmatic young with less exposure to air travel and unaware of potential travel problems. Younger people are more likely to consider adversity an adventure.

Flight anxiety is one of the most debilitating experiences for air travellers. Flight anxieties are common phenomena observed in 10-40 % of air travellers dependent on pre-flight and in-flight situations. [2]This proportion is likely to have increased with the deleterious change in the pre-flight experience and terrorist threat to aircraft. They can result in undesirable consequences. Flight anxiety may predispose passengers to stress-related illnesses and cardiological problems, which may result in-flight emergencies.[3] Apart from potential health damaging effects, it may have an adverse effect on social interaction.[4] Stress of air travel has been found to disrupt passengers' behaviour.[5] Stressed and anxious passengers may become more demanding, dissatisfied and easily agitated in communication with the crew or other passengers. Fatigued and overwrought they can exhibit disruptive behaviour ranging from verbal aggression to severe physical aggression.

Air transport related anxieties may be enhanced in anxiety prone personalities, the vulnerable old and be affected by cultural values and external environmental influences.[6] All shape the subjectively experienced cognitive and emotional impact of the overall flying experience. Airport environments and flights often pose novel situations where personal control is limited and bureaucracy, overt and covert regulation and rules add to frustrations.[7] Attribution of blame and satisfactory redress from front line staff, which might diffuse build-up of stress rarely occurs, as they too have scant control over the predicament. The air travelling public people are reacting to these psychological pressures by changes in behaviour, belatedly being recognised by the transport industry.

Travel related stress in older travellers starts before departure with change from home-established routines. The land journey can be affected by adverse road/rail conditions and the traveller can be stressed by time of arrival at the departure terminal. Stress mounts incrementally with progression through airport security, now a major source of psychological disturbance for passengers. There is invasion of individual privacy with potential embarrassment on the luggage search, enforced taking off of shoes, belts and body frisking. Authoritarian demands of security staff are objectionable and the process an unwelcome reminder that the aeroplane may be blown–up in en route. Restriction on hand luggage is an additive irritant for most travellers, adding to the increasing frustration engendered by passage to the aeroplane. The passenger has been reduced to a mere seat number in an uncaring bureaucratic process. Communication failures are tension-causing when systems collapse under overload. The procedural process is annoying, diminishing and demeaning and added to inevitable flight delays and failures, continued frustration brings increasing stress, tension and aberrant behaviour in airport or the air and physiological change which may endanger health.[6]

In a study undertaken at Heathrow airport in 2007, passengers had heart and finger monitors fitted to record blood pressure and pulse rate while in the airport en- route to flight departure. Skin conductance-a reliable measure of stress- was also measured. Readings were correlated with the amount of psychological stress they experienced.[7 a.b]

Passengers passing through the airport, who were healthy and not exercising, showed monitored stress levels equivalent to on-duty riot police. During the test, there were marked physiological changes. ECG and BP monitors showed immediate and sustained changes:- Within minutes of entering the terminal, heart rates had increased from 55 beats per minute to over 70 per minute in the non-exercising state.

In the average 4 hours it took to board the aircraft, rates continued to rise to more than 200 beats per minute in transit with a rise also occurring in blood pressure.

Queues at check-in and security increased blood pressure levels from average of 123/81 mm Hg to 170/99mm Hg. There was a marked increase in skin conductance with a rise 100 times that in a relaxed state. Associated stress levels peaked four times but were sustained at a high level overall.

Causes of peaking were queues, unfriendly, unhelpful staff, lack of or misinformation Monitoring on the return journey revealed that return transit through the air port was almost as stressful as departure, primarily because of queues at immigration, security channels and lost luggage.

A similar study on passengers travelling by, road and train confirmed the stress felt by delayed passengers .Pulse rate of train passengers increased with the queue for departure and while the train was in the Channel tunnel. Car drivers were stressed on boarding the ferry and adapting to foreign driving. Only coach passenger remained relaxed during travel. [8]

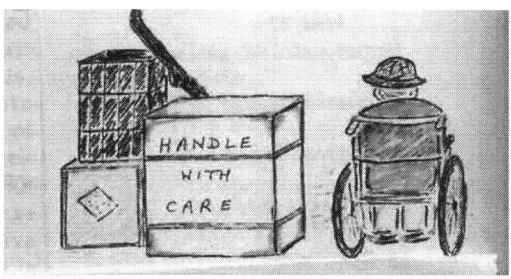

A study of 1009 passengers transiting an airport reported that 69% stated that rude staff were a contributory problem to stress with 52% considering this a major cause of travel related stress.[9] Behavioural responses are also evident with 42% of travellers admitting to repeatedly checking travel documents prior to the flight and international journey, with these obsessive compulsive tendencies greater in women.A third admit they check passports at least five times from arrival at the departure point to boarding, although they do not normally exhibit obsessive behaviour.

Coping strategies for Air Travel Anxieties.

Half of all worried travellers do nothing to minimise their anxieties. Many admit behavioral responses .[10]

Several coping strategies are adopted by passengers for air-travel worries:-
*   9% avoid flying if possible

- 16% use relaxation and distraction techniques
- 13% use alcohol drinking for relaxation in flight
- 6% resort to sedatives

Virgin Atlantic now offers in-flight audio meditation programmes with tips on relaxation from a psychotherapist to help diminish passenger stress. Many travellers resort to cognitive strategies to diminish and deal with the travel experience and affluent older passengers particularly can reduce the effect of adverse circumstances by travelling in first class.[11]

Coping strategies or mechanisms are thinking patterns and cognitive frameworks that individuals use when stressed and aroused, in order to regulate their emotional state and alleviate anxieties Passengers distract themselves by reading, writing, utilising relaxation techniques or other activity which directs attention from flight or pre-flight experience. Music listening can induce calmness. Alcohol, smoking and tranquilliser pills are also used to handle stress.

Younger air travellers are most likely to minimise the seriousness of their flight experience, reflect on personal fears and anxieties over flying and remind themselves of pleasant experience, either relevant or irrelevant to the flight situation, as strategies to cope with current distress. Insistently thinking about the risks of flying, picturing the worst possible scenario to minimise one's fear and blaming other people are the least frequently utilised strategies. However many older people admitted to brooding over worst scene scenarios as day of departure approached.[10]

New coping strategies are being developed in passengers exposed to airport environmental challenge, but they are however limited in potential adaptation manoeuvres. Weight restrictions limit food, drink and pastimes to be taken airside to ameliorate prolonged waiting and make it almost impossible to prepare for prolonged delay or a night or two spent on a departure lounge floor. Maladaptation results in aggressive behaviour and has brought a resultant increase in reported police intervention at major airports.[12]

Passengers are now adopting the classical response to potential stressful situations – avoidance.[11] They are seeking alternative means of reaching destinations. Long distance train companies report increased business with more well used and more trains. Ferry companies to the continent are attracting more travellers. The cruise lines diligently survey regular and potential passengers and they report an increasing demand for UK port to port cruises. The arrival of fly cruising 20 years ago had driven these from the scene, but they are regaining popularity.

Intending passengers approach health professionals for anxiolytics and sleeping pills to reduce travel anxieties but their prescription should be resisted. The latter may result in deep vein thrombosis on long flights due to limb immobility and cognitive behavioural techniques are advised rather than anxiolytics in older people who may already be on other drug medication and risk adverse drug interaction.[13]

The travel health professional should have an understanding of passengers' subjective experiences and anxieties over flying and the use of coping strategies.Adequate knowledge on psychological aspects of air travel and specifics of worry experience, along with anxiety provoking situations should inform management and direct pretravel advice to minimise psychological and physiological stress.

Coping advice for air travellers.

Use alternatives to air transport when possible
Book into airline courtesy lounges.
Travel in best affordable class
Book into local hotel accommodation, the night prior to departure.
Assume delay and take reading material, games, emergency food and water, a ground sheet and small pillow.
Avoid air travel in winter, the strike season and round public holidays.

Flying phobias

Flying phobias and fear of tunnels are common and affect old and young. They can inhibit sufferers from undertaking global travel. With good management, disabling fear, disturbed conditioned responses and frantic avoidance behaviour can be replaced by rational activity.

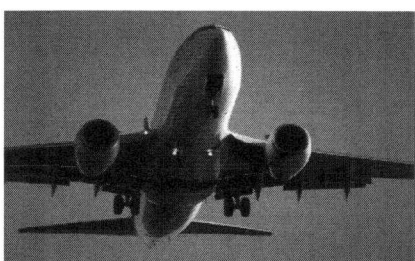

Anticipation and apprehension.
 Typically, the older phobic presents to the family doctor a few days before a long planned flight to a popular holiday resort. Months previously the family have convinced grandmum or dad that they can overcome a reluctance to fly and the vacation is arranged. As the time for departure draws ever closer, apprehension increases with anticipation and shortly before the dread day it becomes apparent to the patient that he or she cannot face the perceived ordeals of an air passage. An acute anxiety state results which reaches crisis proportions as the family becomes teed up for the departure. This presents as a specific phobia which may be associated with panic reaction.[14]
The majority of phobics appear to be women although women may be more likely to report their fears that men. Travel phobias represented 2.81 per cent of phobias reported by women in surveys [15,16] In a 10 per cent random sample of 7,074 patients in general practice based on a structured questionnaire listing 13 common fear-provoking objects or situations, 16 per cent admitted to having a phobia and 13 percent of this sub-group reported fear of flying with a female to male preponderance of 2:1.[17]
 Disproportionate reaction.
Fear is of course a normal and essential condition for everyday living. It is a response to a real or imagined threat with a behavioural element which is often pronounced. Minor fears are within the cultural norm and there is a continuum between mild and intense fears with the latter usually described as phobia. This is *considered a morbid response disproportionate to the causative stimulus.* Sufferers often structure their lives to avoid fear-provoking situations.

In a **Phobia:**

The degree of anxiety and fear is :-

out of all proportion to evoking situation
cannot be explained or reasoned away
beyond voluntary control
leads to avoidance

Definition

The phobic reaction is totally out of proportion to the situational trigger, is involuntary and cannot be explained or reasoned away by the individual involved. It leads to incapacitating avoidance behaviour and it is likely that there are many more people with flying phobias than the statistics suggest, as most simply avoid any likelihood of exposure to air travel. Those with such a condition have an irrational, uncontrollable fear resulting in avoidance behaviour which may disturb their lifestyle.

To understand the phobic's reactions one has to consider the cognitive, physiological and behavioural components involved. The *psychic element* appears as overt anxiety and an exaggerated arousal response when exposed to the feared situation or even consideration of exposure, e.g. as the day of the dreaded flight draws closer. The *physiological response* results in a sweating, tremulous, palpitating and breathless patient with assorted pains from muscle tension. The primeval fight or flight reflexes poorly prepared such people for today's flight demands. *Avoiding behaviour* by the travelling executive or salesman, or the housewife's refusal to contemplate air travel thus depriving her family of a holiday in the sun, introduces a *social element* which often finally forces the patient to seek professional help.

Freudian approach

This model of a phobia helps towards a useful understanding of the problem and provides a practical approach to appropriate therapy. ***The vicious phobic cycle is open to curative intervention at three levels*** through different components.

Relaxation can be taught to control physical symptoms, **cognitive therapy** helps to control and change fear-provoking thoughts and **exposure treatment** can help to overcome the restrictions in lifestyle.

In most cases it is not known how a phobia has developed. Sometimes there is a clear cut trigger such as an unhappy incident occurring on a flight or to an aircraft before or after travel. Some are simply conditioned fear reactions. It is likely that we are more genetically predisposed to make fearful links with some situations and objects than with others; as humans we are phylogenetically prepared to learn certain stimulus responses than alternatives. A Freudian approach to the condition would accept that, when someone shows fear of something he knows to be harmless, then the phobic object or situation is associated with or symbolises something else that is genuinely dangerous. Freud believed that the inner conflict in such a case is then repressed and repressive aspects of it are displaced on to alternative external objects symbolising the repressed complex.

Components occurring in phobic states

Cognitive element – person is subjectively afraid
Behavioural response – avoidance of feared situation
Physiological Manifestation – tachycardia; hyperventilation which often lead to:
A social component – disruption of normal living

Therapeutic approach

Given time, therapy can usually bring alleviation of symptoms and cure and, even at the eleventh hour, patients can be helped towards and along the frightening path from airport to aircraft and on with the flight. A phobia specific to flying can be dealt with most easily but air travel involves more than boarding the aeroplane. Crowded departure lounges will disturb the agoraphobic, the closed inescapable environment of the jet-liner frightens those with a fear of closed spaces, climbing the steps to the doorway of a jumbo jet towering above will upset those with a fear of heights, and the necessity to eat in public will give anxiety to those with a social phobia. All these possibilities must be kept in mind when preparing to treat the patient who wants to make the feared flight and the even more dreaded return.

Approached at the last moment a harassed family physician, battling through a busy surgery, will probably reach for the prescription pad and prescribe a tranquilliser. This hurried response might get the patient on to the aeroplane where, with the added boost of recourse to in-flight duty free alcohol, the flight might just be made tolerable. The prescribed drug does nothing to cure the underlying condition, however, and merely treats the symptoms with the risk of initiating dependence upon anxiolytic drug therapy. Other therapies are available which can usually cure the patient. When drugs are used they ought to be prescribed for the very short term. Benzodiazepines [18] are givem for general anxiety, with higher dosage in anticipation of the phobic event, and the patient advised to refrain from taking alcohol or a hypnotic on the flight. Beta-blockers are used to control peripheral sympathetic responses such as palpitations. In entrenched agoraphobia with travel phobic manifestations there is some evidence that clomipramine has an antiphobic effect but it has to be given in high dosages. Any anti-depressant may well lift a specific phobia which has been a symptom of an underlying depression.

Behaviour modification

Given time before the need to travel, behaviour modification is widely used in clinics to treat phobics.[19] The principal is to expose the patient to the situation which causes distress until he gets used to it and attempts are then made to extinguish the fear by relating it to a pattern of response which provokes no anxiety. The problem behaviour needs detailed study in order to arrive at a hypothesis about its genesis and identify appropriate intervention.

Desensitisation[19] consists of two features; **muscle relaxation and reduction of anxiety and the construction of a graded hierarchy of aversive stimuli** from information provided by the patient. Such a hierarchy for a flying phobia would consist of arrival at the airport, proceeding to the departure lounge, walking on to the plane, experiencing take-off and landing. The hierarchy can be presented to the patient, either in imagery or in reality, and film and tape recordings can be used effectively in desensitisation. Treatment can be assisted by vicarious or participant modelling. Here the therapist approaches the feared object or situation and demonstrates his confident response to it before asking the patient to do likewise. This procedure has three functions; the model encourages new patterns of behaviour to be adopted, unnecessary responses are inhibited or disinhibited and the expression of already established responses can be facilitated.

Desensitisation works well with social and specific phobias and British Airways and several universities and hospitals have run courses for phobic travellers with success. These often culminate in a short flight round the local town to demonstrate to the sufferer that the phobia has been extinguished. The disadvantage is that the process is time-consuming and often requires many sessions. Desensitisation can be carried out, however, with minimal therapist contact using tape recordings and book instruction on relaxation and desensitization procedures.

Hypnosis treatment for phobias [20] borrows both from behaviour modification and desensitization but therapy is facilitated by induction of a trance state.

Teaching the patient auto-hypnosis, whereby at a coded signal he can recreate the relaxed state acquired at earlier sessions, decreases the risk of dependence and diminishes the time required for therapy. Graded desensitisation and flooding are both practicable within the trance states and visual imagery and vicarious modeling can also be used. A modified flooding technique is used and it is very effective for specific phobias such as flying.[21]

Case History

One of my patients, who had patiently built up his business, had a unique opportunity presented to his firm for advancement and profit in the Far East, but he had long had a phobia for air travel. Unable to resist the opportunity for expansion he made his plans, bought his tickets, and the day before departure succumbed to panic and terror at the thought of many hours incarcerated in an aircraft. In the surgery he was in a state of agitation but refused to consider a drug prescription as he wished to be mentally fit for tough business negotiations upon arrival in Hong Kong.

He accepted the offer of hypnotherapy with alacrity and, providing to be good subject, was quickly in a trance and relaxed. Soon he was able to create a visual image of himself boarding and sitting in the aeroplane and, with continued suggestion of calmness, muscle and mind relaxation and freedom from tension, he was able to fantasise himself through a prolonged exposure to the feared situation. Given post-hypnotic suggestions that he would remain calm throughout the flight, and that the standard pre-take off and recorded music would relax him, he went off to make a successful return flight and business deal. Even when the jet-liner was buffeted badly by turbulence and suddenly dropped 500 feet, with the dramatic appearance of personal passenger oxygen masks from their overhead stowage, he was able to keep calm. Now after a decade and many air trips he remains undisturbed by his once disabling phobia.

"Gentle words, quite words are after all the most powerful words. They are more convincing, more compelling, more prevailing and successful," an elderly lady wrote to me on return from her first successful air trip after years of phobic avoidance. However the removal of psychosomatic symptoms before the patient is ready, and has built up more socially satisfactory defences, can precipitate more serious difficulties and therapists have to keep this in mind. It seems likely, however, that desensitisation can be carried out with little therapist contact using tape recordings to carry out relaxation and desensitisation procedures, and these are certainly a useful adjuvant in desensitisation and hypnotherapy. Book and computer instruction courses offering graded and detailed programmes of relaxation and exposure are available, and have proved of value to many phobics.

Conclusion. Although phobias of air travel and flying are common and likely to become more prevalent, the phobic air traveller need not despair as there are thriving phobic societies and several books and many therapists available to proffer support and guidance. With good management, the disabling fear, disturbed conditioned responses and frantic avoidance behaviour can be replaced by rational activity and more normal, socially acceptable reactions and conditioned responses.

BEHAVIOURAL DISTURBANCE

Elderly people are not immune to the behavioural disturbance referred to as air rage. A build up of fatigue, frustration and anger can result in verbal and physically aggressive behaviour to fellow travellers and staff. Over indulgence in alcohol drinking and medication interaction can result in behavioural misconduct and they should be aware of this risk. Alcohol intake on long flights is best avoided by those on routine medication and affected by a measure of kidney failure – a consideration for many older travellers as a third of those over 80 will be affected by grade 3a chronic kidney disease.

Early Alzheimer's disease can be seen in the aberrant behaviour displayed by some elderly vacationers. [13] Sometimes solo travellers they can be seen wandering round cruise ships and getting lost from tour groups. Their fellows are usually tolerant and supportive but they put themselves at health risk on ships and in road traffic. Unaccustomed surroundings and travel related stressors add to their confusional states.

They are particularly likely to become disorientated in airports In 40% of these early cases some measure of agitation, sleep disturbance , wandering increased irritability and aggression are apparent. 13 Locational change tends to increase their mental stability and they should be discouraged from participating in holidays with an ever changing environment such as cruise, coach or, train tour. If they do travel anti-psychotic medication should be reviewed before departure. They should travel with a companion and provisional plans should be in place for unwanted illness in the accompanying person.

Case *History*. *A 75 year old man had travelled alone to Australia despite a diagnosis of senile dementia. His visit to family was successful but on the return, tired, dehydrated and confused he became disturbed and wandered around Heathrow for many hours while transferring aeroplanes. Totally disorientated he missed his onward flight and was only identified as ill and lost by a patrolling policemen, after the last flight of the day had departed. He never fully recovered his former cognitive state and was institutionalised when he finally arrived in his home town*

References

1 McIntosh, Swanson, Power, Fiona, & Dempster, 2006Prevalence,intensity, and sex differences in travel related stressors, Journal of Travel Medicine, 3 (2), 96-102.).

2 McIntosh, Swanson, Power,Raeside & Dempster, 1998. Anxiety and health problems related to air travel, Journal of Travel Medicine, 5 (4), 198-204.

3 Van Gerwen, Spinhoven, Diekstra & Van Dyck, 1997;.People who seek help for fear of flying: Typology of flying phobics, behaviour therapy, 28 (2), 237-25107 9,595,923

4 Bor, 2007. Psychological factors in airline passenger and crew behaviour: A clinical overview. Travel Medicine and Infectious Disease, 5 (4), 207–216.

5 Abubakar and Mavondo, 2002. The determinants of anxiety in air travel: an exploratory study. ANZMAC Conference Proceedings,2741-2747.

6 Cox ID, Blight A, Lyons JP Air-terminal stress and the older traveller Age Ageing. 1999 Mar;28(2):236-7.

7a McIntosh IB 2003 Flying-related stress. In Bor, R. (Ed.),Passenger behaviour (pp. 17-31). Ashgate Publishing:Hampshire.

7b Lewis D. Heathrow stress equal to facing riots.2007.Neuroco International . Travel Telegraph.Aug. 8

8 Milward D. Let the coach take the strain of long distance travel . 2008 Travel telegraph Feb 7 8

9.Kraaij,Garnefski, & van Gerwen, 2003Cognitive coping and anxiety among people with fear flying. In Bor, R. & vanGerwen, L. (Eds.), Psychological Perspectives on Fear of Flying.Ashgate Publishing.

10 Bor, R. (2003).. In Bor, R. (Ed.), Passenger Behaviour Ashgate Publishing

11 McIntosh, I. B. (2003). Flying-related stress. In Bor, R. (Ed.),Passenger behaviour (pp. 17-31). Ashgate Publishing:Hampshire

12 McIntosh I Psychological and behavioural Change in Vacation Air travellers. Travelwise. 2011

13 Connolly P. Dementia management 2011. Ger. Med. 41. Sup 05. 34-40

14 Agras S., Sylvester., and Oliveau D., 196-9. The epidemiology of common fears and phobias. Comprehensive Psychiatry, 10: 2, 151

15 Wilson G., 1967. Social desirability and sex differences in expressed fear. Behaviour research and therapy, 5: 136.

16 Burns L., Thorpe G., 1977. Fears and phobias. Journal of international Medical Research, 5: Suppl. 1: 132-139.

17 France R., Robson M., 1986. Behaviour therapy in primary care 66. Croom Helm Publishers.

18 Tyrer P., 1989. Treating Panic. British Medical Journal, 298: 201.

19 McIntosh I., 1980. Incidence, management and treatment of phobias in a group medical practice. Pharmaceutical Medicine 1, 2: 77-82

20 France R., Robson M., 1986. Behaviour therapy in primary care 66. Croom Helm Publishers.

21 McIntosh I., 1981. Hypnotherapy: The case for the GP. Psychiatry in Practice, November 1981.

Iain B. McIntosh

Chapter 10

Infection and Disease in Older people.

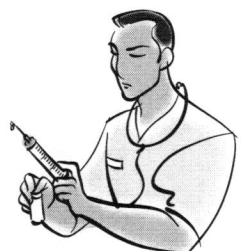

Immunisation

The ageing of populations in developed countries has greatly increased the number of older world traveller, with estimates of 13% of travellers being at least 65 years old. Five to 8% of travellers in tropical areas are old persons. Immunisations are recommended for older people because age generally aggravates the impact of infectious diseases and they often have chronic medical conditions. The immune system deteriorates in old age. especially where immune response is dependent upon cellular immunity and humoural response. The number and functions of T-lymphocytes decrease, but B-lymphocytes are not altered. The response to vaccinations is therefore slower and lower in efficacy in the elderly. Reduced ability to seroconvert is attributed to immune-senescence. This has multiple elements and is difficult to measure. It includes T cell reduction from thymic involution, less effective antigen presentation through monocytes, and reduced killer cell toxicity.[1]

Vaccination requirements for older travellers are broadly similar to younger people except that additional factors have to be considered. Loss of immunity, the effect of routine medications and seroconversion after vaccination are relevant in this group. People going on trips involving travel in confined spaces with other travellers , such as bus trips and cruise ships, are at additional risk as are older people with reduced immunity ,such as those with HIV, taking high dose long-term steroids or receiving chemotherapy. Another complicating factor is that older travellers may often have a vague knowledge of past immunization records and infectious diseases

Older adults are especially vulnerable to certain diseases, such as influenza and pneumonia. In 2008, adults aged 65 and older comprised 90 percent of deaths that occur every year from complications related to influenza and pneumonia. Pneumonia is a major cause of morbidity and mortality in elderly people, especially in those with chronic medical conditions such as chronic heart and lung diseases. Influenza is another prime cause of death in old people.

Influenza, pneumococcal, zoster, tetanus, poliomyelitis, hepatitis and typhoid fever vaccinations are commonly recommended for senior citizens before world travel. The effects of age diminished immunity response are observed with vaccinations against tetanus, flu, pneumococcal infections and hepatitis B.2

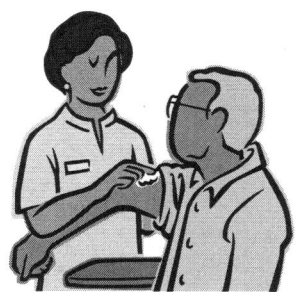

Influenza

Influenza and pneumonia are responsible for about 8% of all deaths in old people, with influenza being the 4th commonest cause of death after cancer, heart disease and stroke. There is limited evidence of benefit of the influenza vaccine in the over-65s from Randomised Controlled Trials (RCTs). However, cohort studies suggest that those who are vaccinated do seem to fare better in terms of reduced hospital admissions and total mortality, The evidence for benefit is sufficiently strong that influenza vaccine is recommended throughout Europe. The success of the vaccine depends upon seroconversion in the individual, and then the extent to which the strain in the vaccine matches the circulating viral strain. Seroconversion after vaccination occurs in, 60% of community-dwelling subjects around 60 30% in 70-80's, and 12% in those over 80. Annual influenza vaccination is recommended for those over 65 years age and should be offered to all global older travellers if they have not been protected. The seroconversion, after vaccine, is 50% from 60 to 70 years old, 31% from 70 to 80 years old, and only 11% after 80 years old. Vaccination reduces morbidity by 25%, admission to hospital by 20%, pneumonia by 50%, and mortality by 70%. 1-3.4-8

Pneumonia

Pneumococcal disease is caused by the bacterium Streptococcus resulting in pneumonia, meningitis and septicaemia which can be life-threatening. Vaccination is recommended for older adults over 65 year's age because as they are more vulnerable to infection. Pneumococcal vaccine is effective in 60% of older recipients. Pneumococcal vaccine is indicated every five years for those over 65 years of age or with chronic diseases and post-splenectomy. The 23-valent Pneumococcal polysaccharide vaccine is used in most European countries for adults aged over 60 yrs and is particularly indicated for those with asplenia, are immunocompromised, have chronic cardiac, renal, pulmonary or liver disease, and recipients of organ transplants. Meta-analysis has shown a 36% reduction in pneumococcal pneumonia, but no overall effect on pneumonia mortality .8The efficacy varies with the age of the population studied and the endpoint used: in adults aged 65-74 years, the vaccine is 70-80% effective, falling to 53-67% in 75-84 yr olds, and even further to 0-22% in the group aged 85 yrs and above. 1.2

Tetanus

Tetanus is fatal in 32% of the people above 80 years, therefore this vaccination is important. Adults are now recommended to have a tetanus booster at age 50 unless they have had a booster in the previous 10 years.

Diptheria

Diphtheria is caused by the bacterium Corynebacterium diphtheriae, which infects the upper respiratory tract. A grey membrane may form in the throat and obstruct breathing. The bacteria also produce a toxin that may affect nerves and the heart.Adults are recommended to have a diphtheria booster vaccination at age 50 unless they have had a booster in the previous 10 years. Diphtheria and tetanus boosters are usually combined in one injection.

Shingles

Herpes zoster is caused by the chickenpox virus, (varicella-zoster). When infected for the first time, it causes chickenpox but the virus stays in the nerve cells, where it is kept in check by the immune system. With age, the immune system is less effective, the virus may be reactivated and cause shingles. Older people may develop complications of shingles with enduring pain, or the rash may spread to the eye. A vaccine for herpes zoster was licensed in 2006 in Europe for immune-competent adults aged 60 or over, and recommendations amended to include adults over 50 yrs in 2007.The use of herpes zoster vaccine reduced the incidence by 51 percent, incidence of post-herpetic neuralgia by 66 percent, and the overall burden of illness due to zoster by 61 percent 9The vaccine has uncertain duration of benefit, and the severity of post-herpetic neuralgia is greater above 70 years.

Vaccination against zoster is recommended for adults aged 60 and over, unless they have already received a dose of zoster vaccine, are allergic to any of its ingredients or have another disease, or treatment that significantly lowers their immunity. Only one dose of zoster vaccine is needed. 9

Hepatitis A virus

(HAV) exposure in unprotected adults may cause severe and serious symptoms, with risk of both morbidity and mortality increasing with age. With hepatitis A, there has also been shown to be an association between an age of >40 years of age and severe morbidity and high mortality: the mortality rate is 2.5% for patients who are >40 years of age, compared with a rate of <0.1% among younger patients.

As seroprevalence of HAV is low in industrialised countries, and an increasing number of elderly people, travel from areas of low HAV endemicity to high endemicity, pre-travel vaccination is warranted. Vaccination of the elderly against HAV, , may be associated with reduced seroprotection, since the immune response decreases with age. Studies with monovalent hepatitis A vaccine or combined hepatitis A and B vaccine show good efficacy in adults in general. Administering monovalent hepatitis A vaccine in the elderly showed a reduced seroprotection of approximately 65% after a single primary dose in subjects over the age of 50 years. Seroprotection was 98% in this age group after receiving a booster dose. Giving combined hepatitis A and B vaccine in those older than 40 years showed similar seroprotection (99-100%) against HAV compared to a monovalent vaccine after receiving three doses .Based on available data, travel health professionals should screen elderly travellers to areas endemic for HAV for the presence of naturally acquired immunity, and, if found susceptible, immunise well in advance of their trip, to allow time for post-vaccination antibody testing and/or administration of a second dose of the vaccine.[10]

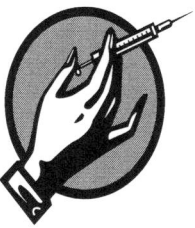

Poliomyelitis

Naturally acquired anti-poliovirus immunity does not seem to decrease with age, unlike anti-diphtheria and anti-tetanus immunity.

Tuberculosis

The tuberculin skin test is an easy method to check risk in elderly people. A negative result indicates depressed cell-mediated immunity.

Yellow fever

Older travellers (those aged over 60 years) who have not previously been vaccinated against yellow fever are at a higher risk of side effects with the yellow fever vaccine. Serious adverse reactions to immunisation increase from I in 250,000 to 1 in50,000 in over-sixties in people not immunised previously. [11-14]

Malaria

Malaria is one of the most prevalent global diseases, with an infected population of 300–500 million and 1.5–3.5 million deaths reported annually. The major killer is Plasmodium falciparum, which causes multi-organ involvement and, in the absence of prompt and appropriate treatment, is associated with high mortality rates. Extensive advice on the correct use of exposure- and chemoprophylaxis of malaria is especially important for travellers above the age of 60.Old age is a risk factor for complications of malaria in the non-immune traveller with higher risk for a severe course of malaria in the elderly. There is significant evidence for a correlation between age and the frequency of complications in malaria such as cerebral involvement, respiratory failure, renal failure, anaemia, and hyper-parasitaemia.

- In patients over 15 years of age, 37.1 % developed a severe course of malaria, whereas in those 60 years and above this percentage increased to 61.5 %.
- The age distribution in the group with severe malaria was significantly shifted towards the elderly (p = 0.016 in Mann-Whitney test).
- The duration of hospitalisation also increased with age from an average of five days for the group below 45 years to 21 days for the elderly of 60 years and above.[15,16]

In a national Israeli analysis of P. falciparum malaria in non-immune patients, there was a significantly higher rate of severe disease and mortality among those patients who were over 40 years of age](16) In an Indonesian study, mortality from malaria was highest in the youngest (<2 years) and oldest age groups (>40 years), 2.2% and 2.5%, respectively, compared with 0%–0.9% for patients who were 2–40 years of age. [17]

In patients who died of imported P. falciparum malaria in 1959–1987 in the United States. A breakdown of the study population by age groups showed that there was an increment in mortality by age: in the 0–19-, 20–39-, 40–69-, and 70–79-year-old age groups, the case fatality rates were 0.4%, 2.2%, 5.8%, and 30.3%, respectively.[18]Other studies show similar results. The number of severe cases increased with age 3.2% of cases in patients who were <30 years of age; 5.3%, for patients 30–39 years of age; 9.8%, for patients 40–49 years of age; and 23.5%, for patients ≤50 years of age. [19]Sabatinelli et al [20] showed a 2.3% case fatality rate in patients with malaria due to P. falciparum, with increment in mortality by age .Mortality rate was 0.5% in patients 21–30 years of age; 2.3%, in patients 31–40 years of age; 1.7%, in patients 41–50 years of age; and 5.4%, in patients ≤51 years of age.

These studies included a mixed population of non immune travellers and immigrants, and all examined different end points (either severity or mortality of malaria). Age (over 40 years) is the most important risk factor for predicting severe malaria, In 5 studies with a total of 4146 patients who had malaria due to P. falciparum a case fatality rate of 1.1% among the patients who were <40 years of age, compared with 5.3% in patients who were ≤40 years of age. [19,20]

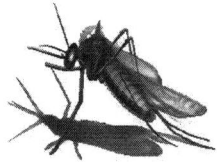

The reason for the increased vulnerability at the age of more than 40 years age is not clear. One explanation may be the underlying medical conditions of the aged patients. Baird [16] hypothesized,that different immune responses that are related to age may be responsible for the different outcomes. The susceptibility of the aged population to the negative effect of cytokines excreted during the disease may be higher. Older persons may use prophylaxis less than did younger patients (~79% of the elderly patients did not take any prophylaxis, compared with 52% of the younger patients) in one study. Complete prophylaxis was taken by only 2% of the older patients, whereas 10% of the younger patients took complete prophylaxis. These findings may not be generalizable , but, if so, may explain the higher attack rate in the elderly population.[17]

Many senior citizens have chronic medical conditions and are on a multiplicity of medications which can interact with antimalarial prophylaxis,which can complicate preventive interventions. For instance some antimalarials lower insulin requirements in diabetic patients and can lead to hypoglycaemia in those treated with insulin or oral hypoglycaemics such as glibenclamide. Both chloroquine and mefloquine also have the potential to increase the risk of arrhythmias if given with other antiarrythmic agents such as amiodarinei.It is best to avoid a range of cardioactive drugs including beta blockers, antiarrythmics and calcium antagonsists in combination with mefloquine. This is due to the risk of prolonging the QTc interval and inducing other cardiac adverse effects.(see chap.7)

Recommendations

- Clinicians should provide aged travellers with specific instructions for prophylaxis of malaria, encourage complete compliance, and vigorously treat patients when they show the first clinical signs of malaria.
- Medical history, current medications and decreased immunity status have to be considered.
- Recommendations should be based on individualised, customised analysis of infection risk with a review of travel venue, prevalence of malaria in the area and whether p.vivax or p.falciparum is locally endemic and whether exposure is continuous or sporadic.

- Concise risk appraisal is mandatory to provide the traveller with accurate information on personal risk while exposed to mosquito bites on a short vacation. Global travel in this group is frequently in city and urban areas with exposure only during daytime hours. Many aged tourists are only exposed to the local environment on day time coach tours and will spend much of their time in air conditioned buildings and coaches with minimal exposure to biting mosquitos. Passengers on cruises visiting endemic areas will often be off shore at dusk and during the night and daytime exposure will be limited.
- The health professional should consider whether the risk of serious side effects from prophylactic medication may be greater than the risk of acquiring the disease.
- The need for barrier prevention of bites needs to be emphasised with the wearing of trousers and long sleeved garments and the repeated application of insect repellent containing DEET. [21]

PROPHYLAXIS

No reduction in antimalarial dosage is required on the basis of advanced age. However, elderly travellers are more likely to have underlying disorders, for example renal or liver impairment, which may necessitate antimalarial dose reduction. The increased likelihood of elderly travellers taking additional medication, for chronic conditions, will influence choice of chemo-prophylactic agent. [22]

Chloroquine, Proguanil, Chloroquine plus proguanil, Mefloquine, Doxycyclin may be appropriate. All have potential side effects and their use has to be carefully considered if there is chronic disorder and the traveller is on routine medication. [21-26]

Drug interactions

Proguanil may enhance the anticoagulant effect of warfarin a medication commonly taken in older patients. Mefloquine antagonises the anticonvulsant effect of antiepileptics and interacts with a number of cardiac drugs. Mefloquine prophylaxis is contraindicated in those with current, or previous history of depression, neuro-psychiatric disorders or epilepsy; or with hypersensitivity to quinineThe metabolism of doxycycline is accelerated by carbamazepine andphenytoin. [2,27]

Travellers needing malaria chemoprophylaxis and currently taking warfarin:

- Tetracyclines possibly enhance the anticoagulant effect of coumarins (e.g. warfarin),• Travellers should start taking antimalaria tablets more than 1 week(and ideally 2-3 weeks in the case of mefloquine) prior to their departure.
- A baseline INR should be checked prior to starting chemoprophylaxis, and re-checked after 1 week of taking chemoprophylaxis.
- If a traveller is away for a long period of time the INR should be checked at intervals at the destination. Once chemoprophylaxis has been completed, the INR should be checked again to re-stabilise anticoagulant therapy.

Liver disease

Most antimalarial drugs are excreted or metabolised by the liver with a risk of drug accumulation in severe liver impairment.

- In severe liver disease: all antimalarial drugs are contraindicated, with the possible exception of atovaquone plus proguanil.
- For moderate impairment: proguanil, or atovaquone plus proguanil or mefloquine may be used.
- In mild impairment: chloroquine, or proguanil, or chloroquine plus proguanil, or atovaquone plus proguanil or mefloquine may be used. Doxycycline should be used only with caution.

The choice of chemoprophylaxis should be made after discussion with the hepatic specialist, The Child-Pugh classification s often used for grading liver function (accessible at http://www.emea.europa.eu/pdfs/human/ewp/233902en.pdf

Renal impairment

Chloroquine is partially excreted via the kidneys while proguanil is wholly excreted via the kidneys. • Chloroquine: dose reduction for prophylaxis is required only in severe renal impairment.• Proguanil: should be avoided, or the dose reduced .Atovaquone/proguanil is not recommended for patients with a creatinine clearance of less than30mL/minute [28]. Doxycycline or mefloquine may be used in severe renal failure.

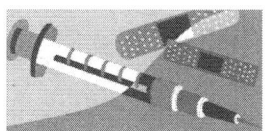

Alternative medications are being explored and vaccination possibilities researched. The therapeutic efficacy of new products such as artemesinin, the active ingredient of the plant artemisia in killing parasites has been established.Consideration is now being given to management change in selected travellers to lower risk areas being given antimalarial testing kits to be taken if fever intervenes. IF the blood tests positive for infection, an antimalarial medication such as artemisinin would then be taken to abort the infection. The drug has few side effects and this may prove a useful management route for the elderly traveller, particularly if they have concomitant medical conditions and are on several routine medications. Cruise passengers in particular making an occasional visit to a malarial area in day time might consider this an option. With compliance an issue in this group, good mechanical barrier protection and prompt treatment when necessary may avoid prophylactic side effects a greater risk to the individual than the chance bite from an infected mosquito[28-30] This approach would depend upon appraisal of risk, provision of adequate information, medication and testing kits to the individual traveller and rely on their compliance and efficient follow-up on UK return.[29,30]

Advice on adequate bite prevention malaria symptoms and prompt treatment with a product like newly licensed artemesinin rather than prophylactic intervention response may be considered.This may be appropriate for non adventurous,elderly seniors on short trips abroad, living in air conditioned rooms in city centres, who are not going on safari, up country, or are living on board ship overnight and are likely to be poorly compliant in taking prophylactic medication.Their actual exposure to mosquitos may be minimal and adverse reactions to antimalarial medication can present a higher risk than malarial infection.Renal and hepatic impairment concomitant with ageing, in the elderly traveller with pre-existing illness,on medications and drug interactions may slant the risk assessment towards non drug malarial recommendations.This response depends upon, thorough history taking , knowledge of travel itinerary, patient's awareness of exposure risk, the need for active personal response to malaria symptoms and their ability to do a blood test and promptly treat with antimalarial medication if tested positive.

Other Infections

Sedentary, non-adventurous, elderly world travellers living in hotels and participating in coach tours may be less likely to acquire infections which often affect the more adventurous young. However the senior citizen sitting by lake or seaside, having a picnic in a forest and overnighting in a hotel can be exposed to insect bites, skin trauma and prolonged healing. Ageing brings lowered immunity, impaired peripheral circulation, poorer skin repair and ankle oedema from cardiac conditions which often result in adverse reaction to minor afflictions. Bites from insects even when not threatening systemic disease can be troublesome. These are a serious threat to diabetic and immuno-compromised elderly travellers. Simple bites from ticks, bed bugs, lice, fleas and sand flies may result in more than a short lasting localised itch, with potential for skin breakdown, ulceration and a lengthy healing process.

Bed bugs (Cimicidae). have increased in prevalence and show increasing resistance to pesticides. They can inhabit top quality hotels and bite bed sleepers. They are small parasitic insects feeding on human blood and are mainly active at night ,biting mainly on legs and feet. They feed unnoticed on hosts, but bites become intensely itchy and can cause skin rashes and allergic symptoms. The itch encourages scratching and excoriation. If there is swelling of the ankles, as often occurs in travellers and those with cardiac problems, or the limb is oedematous, then sores and ulcers can develop. [31]

Treatment is symptomatic. Clean bites with antiseptic and elevate the leg if there is oedema. A topical antihistamine cream will diminish the itch, but the bites create lumps in the skin which continue to itch and can take several weeks to resolve.

Fleas are insects of the order Siphonaptera which are wingless insects with mouthparts adapted for piercing skin and sucking blood. They are external parasites, living by hematophagy off the blood of mammals such as cats, dogs and humans.The wingless insects have tube-like mouth-parts adapted to feeding on the blood of hosts. They move through hairs, or feathers, or, under clothing. The tough flea body is able to withstand great pressure and even hard squeezing between fingers is normally insufficient to kill a flea. They can be eliminated by rolling briskly between the fingers to disable them and crushing then between fingernailso or by direct contact with anti-flea pesticides. Their bites are itchy, and when scratched can become infected and be a problem on swollen limbs.

Treatment. Clean bites with antiseptic and apply topical antihistamine cream.

Sandflies are a species of flying, biting, blood-sucking Dipteran encountered in sandy areas. Their bites leave large, red itchy bumps that may turn into a rash. These bumps are often more itchy ten mosquito bites, and tend to last longer. Some sandfly genera of the Phlebotominae subfamily are primary vectors of leishmaniasis and pappataci fever; both confusingly referred to as sandfly fever. In the New World, leishmaniasis is spread by sand flies. Belize and Honduras are notorious in the Caribbean for sandfly populations.

Prevention and treatment. Tourists to sandy areas should carry bug spray containing high concentrations of DEET and apply antiseptic cream to the bites.

Biting midges. Ceratopogonidae, are a family of small flies (1–4 mm long) in the order Diptera. They are closely related to the Chironomidae, Simuliidae (or black flies), and are found in almost any aquatic or semiaquatic habitat throughout the world.Many are pests in beach or mountain habitats. The blood-sucking species may be vectors of disease-causing viruses, protozoa, and filarial worms. In humans, their bite can cause intensely itchy, red welts that can persist for more than a week. The discomfort arises from a localized allergic reaction to the proteins in their saliva, which can be somewhat alleviated by topical antihistamines. They are notorious for the multiplicity of their bites and intensity of itch produced and are particularly prevalent in the Scottish Highlands and northern latitudes of Scandinavia.

Prevention and treatment. Use of fine screen head veils and spray containing high concentrations of DEET and application of antiseptic cream to bites.

Louse Infestation with Pediculus humanus capitis (head louse) occurs worldwide, and is hyperendemic in many third world populations. [32]Tourists travelling in close contact with indigenous natives in crowded buses, trains and markets in Africa, Asia and South America can become infested. Transmission route is by head to head contact. Pruritus- an immune mediated reaction to components of lice saliva- is the common symptom and may interfere with sleep. Typically, there are reddish, intensely itchy papules, frequently in the retro-auricular area of the scalp. Left untreated this becomes intensely irritating and skin infections may occur if bites are scratched with excoriation.[32].

Treatment methods

There are no functional head lice repellents.

Chemical – Pediculicides containing insecticide with neurotoxic actionare used but are not effective against eggs younger than 4 days age. Increasing resistance is occurring. Topical insecticides –commonly pyrethroids and organophosphatès are used but insecticide resistance is a problem worldwide.[33] They should not be used on broken, secondarily infected skin. Published results cf Cochrane Review ,found no evidence that any one pediculicide has greater effect than another.[34]

Pyrethroids have a a knock-down effect. Permethrin can kill during application and also has a long term residual effect. Most adverse reactions are local and mild. Evidence of efficacy only applies to permethrin 1%.[35]

Organophospates. Malathion inhibits acetylcholinesterase causing louse death by hyper-excitability and exhaustion. It is safe if pure, but needs 20 minutes of application. It can cause skin irritation and asthma attacks.[36]

Herbal Pediculicides containing herbal oils are unproven in efficacy.

Mechanical -Hair combing to remove eggs and lice.

Physical - by means of suffocation. Non-traditional products that contain cyclomethicone or dimeticone work by coating the lice and kill them physically.The potential hazards of pediculicides with neurotoxic action has encouraged development of non-traditional (non-chemical) products that contain cyclomethicone, or dimeticone. These work by coating the lice and killing them physically, by suffocation. Dimeticone (92%) has been produced as a pump spray with one dose action which suffocates lice, larvae and eggs. It has a physical mode of action, low surface tension, is free of chemical insecticide, chemically inert and not absorbed by skin cr mucosae. The substance creeps deeply into the tracheal system of the louse and replaces the air. The volatile dimeticone vaporises, thickens and seals the tubes irreversibly and suffocates all 3 stages of development of nymphs, larvae and eggs. Lice do not appear to become resistant but treatment should be repeated after seven days.[36]

Ticks are small arachnid external parasites, living on the blood of mammals, birds and by default humans. Ticks are vectors of a number of diseases, including Lyme disease,(Lyme borreliosis) and tick-borne encephalitis (TBE).Tick-borne illnesses are caused by infection with a variety of pathogens, including rickettsia and other types of bacteria, viruses, and protozoas.The bite can be anywhere but is often on the legs and thighs. It is initially painless, but after about 36 hours, the site begins to itch and the arachnid may be seen with its head buried in the skin once it has started feeding. If the tick is removed within the first 48 hours of contact then the risk of infection is low. If a herald patch develops around the bite site some days later, Lyme disease has to be considered and treatment with a tetracycline instituted. Doctors and nurses often miss the diagnosis and fail to appreciate the significance of the bites. Older travellers visiting rural areas and spending time in public spaces such as picnic spots, parks and gardens are at risk from tick bites with a high prevalence in northern Europe in vacation months of July and August.

*Treatment.*Embedded Ixodidae should be removed mechanically with forceps and every effort made to ensure the tick's head and mouthparts are not left attached to the person after removal.The site should then be swabbed with an antiseptic cream.

Rabies is a virus infection of mammals transmitted to humans when the skin barrier is breached by bite or scratch, usually by a rabid dog. The older traveller with lowered immune status is vulnerable and should avoid contact with animals in countries where rabies is present. All mammal,bites, scratches and licks on broken skin should be treated immediately with cleaning and antiseptic and consideration given to tetanus booster and rabies vaccination.

References

1 Bourée Immunity and immunization in elderly. P.Pathol Biol (Paris). 2003 Dec;51(10):581-5.

2 Rey M. How to manage vaccinations in the elderly traveller .Bull Soc Pathol Exot. 1997;90(4):245-52.

3.Goodwin K et al Antibody response to influenza vaccination in the elderly: a quantitative review. Vaccine 2006;24:1159-69.

4.Michel J-P et al., Advocating vaccination of adults aged 60 years and older in Western Europe – Rejuvenation Research 2009;12(2):127-136.

6.Potter JM, O'Donnel B Serological response to influenza vaccination and nutritional and functional status of patients in geriatric longterm care. Age Ageing 1999;28:141-5.

7.Mangtani P, Cumberland P, Hodgson CR, et al. A cohort study of the effectiveness of influenza vaccine in older people, performed using the United Kingdom general practice research database. J Infect Dis 2004;190:1–10.

8.Jefferson T, Rivetti D, Rivetti A et al. Efficacy and effectiveness of influenza vaccines in elderly people: a systematic review. Lancet 2005;366:1165-74.

9.Michel J-P et al., Advocating vaccination of adults aged 60 years and older in Western Europe – Rejuvenation Research 2009;12(2):127-136.

10 Genton B, D'Acremont V, Furrer HJ, Hatz C, Louis Loutan Hepatitis A vaccines and the elderly.Travel Med Infect Dis. 2006 Dec;4(6):303-12. Epub 2005 Nov 28.

11 Immunisation against infectious disease - 'The Green Book', Dept of Health (various dates)

12 WHO: Yellow fever vaccine safety, as in Weekly Epidemiological Record (WER) 7 January 2005

13 Lindsey NP, Schroeder BA, Miller ER, et al; Adverse event reports following yellow fever vaccination. Vaccine. 2008 Nov 11;26(48):6077-82. Epub 2008 Sep 20. [abstract]

14 Roukens AH, Visser LG; Yellow fever vaccine: past, present and future. Expert Opin Biol Ther. 2008 Nov;8(11):1787-95.

15 Stich A, Zwicker M, Steffen T, Köhler B, Fleischer K: [Old age as risk factor for complications of malaria in non-immune travellers]. Dtsch Med Wochenschr; 2003 Feb 14;128(7):309-14

16 Baird JK, Masbar S, Basri H, Tirtokusumo S, Subianto B, Hoffman SL. Age-dependent susceptibility to severe disease with primary exposure to Plasmodium falciparum. J Infect Dis 1998;178:592-5.

17. Eli Schwartz, Siegal Sadetzki, Havi Muradand David Raveh Age as a Risk Factor for Severe Plasmodium falciparum Malaria in Nonimmune Patients

18 Greenberg AE, Lobel HO. Mortality from Plasmodium falciparum malaria in travelers from the United States, 1959 to 1987. Ann Intern Med 1990;113:326-7.

19 Calleri G, Lipani F, Macor A, Belloro S, Riva G, Caramello P. Severe and complicated falciparum malaria in Italian travelers. J Travel Med 1998;5:39-41.

20 Sabatinelli G, Majori G, D'Ancona F, Romi R. Malaria epidemiological trends in Italy. Eur J Epidemiol 1994;10:399-403.

21 World Health Organization International travel and health. World Health Organization, G Geneva, 2005.

22 Chiodini P, Hill D, Lalloo D, Lea G, Walker E, Whitty C and Bannister B.Guidelines for malaria prevention in travellers from the United Kingdom. London, Health Protection Agency, January 2007.

23 Meier CR, Wilcock K, Jick SS. The risk of severe depression, psychosis organic attacks with prophylactic antimalarials. Drug Safety.2004; 27:203-13.

24 Wells TS, Smith TC, Smith B et al.Mefloquine use and hospitalizations among US service members, 2002-2004. American Journal of Tropica lMedicine & Hygiene. 2006;74:744-9.

25 Taylor WR, White NJ. Antimalaria ldrug toxicity: a review. Drug Safety.2004;27, 25-61.

26 Ohrt, C, Richie TL, Widjaja H et al.Mefloquine compared with doxycycline for the prophylaxis ofmalaria in Indonesian soldiers .A randomized, double-blind ,placebo-controlled trial. Annals ofInternal Medicine. 1997;126:963-72.

27 Bryant SG, Fisher S, Kluge RM.Increased frequency of doxycycline side effects. Pharmacotherapy.1987;7:125-9.

28 Blackwood T Malaria old and new .2011 J.Brit. Trav health Assoc xvi 2011 34-5

29 World Health Organization. The use of malaria rapid diagnostic tests.2004. World Health Organization.

29 Jelinek T, Grobusch MP, Nothdurft HD.Use of dipstick tests for the rapid diagnosis of malaria in non-immune travelers. Journal of Travel Medicine.2000;7:175-9.

30 Valecha N Phyio P. Mayxay M Randomised study of dihydroartemisinin v. srtensusnate-mefloquine for falciparum malaria in Asia PLoS ONE 2010 5..

31 Melrose A. Bedbugs and bites. 2010 Brit.Trav. Health Assoc. J 15. 24-5

32McIntosh I Louse infestation in Travellers 2011. Brit.trav. heralth Assoc. J. 16.45-7

33 Heukelbach J Management and control of head lice infestations 2010Unined Verlag AD Bremen

34.Cochrane Database Syst Rev. 2001 andCochrane Database Syst Rev. 2000 (2)CD001165

35.Picollo MI.Vassenna Cv et al. Resistance to insecticides and and effect of synergistson permethrin activity in pediculosis capitis.J.Med. E6tomol.2000.37.721-25

36 Gao GR.Yoon KS et al Esterase mediated malathion in the human head louse. Pestic. Biocham. Physiol.200685.28-37

37 Ricchling I Bocleler W. 2008 Lehtal effects of a treatment with dimeticone on insects –Insights in to physical mechanisms. Arzneimitelforshung 58. (5) 248-54

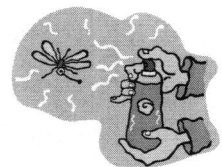

Vaccination and Malaria Prophylaxis Resources

- Travax   www.travax.nhs.uk

- Nathnac   wwwww.nathnac.nhs.uk

- Guidelines for Malaria Prevention in UK Travellers, HPA, Jan 2007 : www.hpa.org.uk

- Immunisation against infectious disease - 'The Green Book' : www.dh.gov.uk

- Health Information for Overseas Travel – 'The Yellow Book' , Nathnac

- International Travel and Health : www.who.int/ith/en/index.html

- CDC Health Information for International Travel 2010 'TheYellow Book' : www.cdc.gov

- The British Society for Rheumatology. Vaccination in the immunocompromised person, guidelines for the patient taking immune suppressants, steroids and the new biologic therapies, 2002:ww.rheumatology.org.uk/includes/documents/cm_docs/2009/v/vaccinations_in_the_im munocompromised_person.pdf

Julie Gallagher. Iain B.McIntosh

Chapter 11.

Travel Medications and Interactions

A number of pharmacological interventions may be made to prepare the traveller going overseas, which include immunisation, malaria chemoprophylaxis and medication for self-treatment, included in a medical kit. Issues related to immunisation are dealt with in chapter ten.

This chapter considers the range of medications that may be prescribed or purchased by the elderly traveller. There are four important principles for consideration:

1.   Is the prescribed medication likely to interact with other medication taken for chronic conditions. Poylpharmacy is common in elderly people, so a medication history should always be sought at consultation.(See chap.1)

2.   Is the medication prescribed for travel likely to be contraindicated? Again the elderly person is more likely to suffer multiple pathologies than a younger individual.(See chap.2)

3.   Is the way that the drug is handled by the body (Pharmacokinetics) likely to be affected in older age e.g. declining liver or renal function. (See chap 1.)

4.   Do much older people tend to respond differently when compared to a younger population (Pharmacodynamics).

?Other points are also worth considering when preparing the traveller who will be carrying any form of medication:

•   Carrying medications across international borders can meet restrictions even when intended for personal use. This particularly applies to those which are designated narcotic or psychotropic drugs. As a rule of thumb, this would cover any medicine that has an effect on the central nervous system and in particular if it could potentially be abused. Carrying a prescription or note from the prescriber and keeping the medication in its original packaging is advocated, but there are some countries, such as the United Arab Emirates, where a range of medicines is completely banned.

•   Adherence to medication may be affected due to a change and disruption in routines whilst away from home.

•   It is always advisable for medications to be purchased before leaving home rather than relying on a local supply even if this is much cheaper. It is estimated that in some countries of Africa and Asia, up to 60% of medicines are counterfeit and many locally produced medicines are of poor quality.Each of the common drugs prescribed in the elderly for travel will be discussed with consideration to these four principles.

First,a brief review of the principles that influence Pharmacokinetics and Pharmacodynamics in old people. [1,2]

Medication Handling in elderly people.

The subject of drug handling is usually considered under headings with the mnemonic ADME; *absorption, distribution, metabolism and excretion*. Also of particular relevance to the elderly are *changes in drug response due to general declining homeostatic mechanisms*.

Absorption of drugs by the gastrointestinal tract is not particularly impaired in the elderly. Gastric Ph tends to be slightly higher in older people but there is no particular evidence that this makes them more prone to travellers' diarrhoea. It is worth bearing in mind that, conditions such as heart failure can potential reduce blood flow to the GIT and thus affect absorption. Drugs with anticholinergic properties such as hyoscine can also potentially reduce drug absorption.

Distribution of drugs around the body can be influenced by the higher proportion of fat and lower proportion of water in the body composition of the elderly person. Further, reduced drug binding to plasma albumin can markedly alter the pharmacokinetics of certain drugs. It is beyond the scope of this chapter to describe the consequences of this in detail, but it can contribute to changes in drug response. One particularly important change in distribution is that drugs tend to cross the blood barrier more readily in the elderly. Thus any drug with potential CNS side effects may be more likely to cause an undesirable outcome and such medication should be prescribed with greater caution. In general, a decline in regional blood flow due to a fall of cardiac output with ageing can reduce the response in target tissues.

Metabolism of drugs.This is decline in blood flow is the major factor contributing to a lower ability to metabolise certain drugs by the liver in the elderly leading to an increased half-life. Other drugs are affected by the decline in liver enzyme activity sometimes manifesting as a reduced first pass affect.

Excretion of drugs by the kidney is also impaired with advancing age, due to the decline in renal function, again manifested by an increased half-life of certain drugs. These affects are particularly important in the presence of extremes of liver/renal dysfunction, or failure.

One important contributor to the general observation that the elderly are more prone to the adverse effects of drugs is the decline in homeostatic mechanisms. For instance the elderly are more prone to postural hypertension which is exacerbated by prescribing any medication that can lower blood pressure. Another example of a potential travel scenario might be, the elderly person taking an ACE inhibitor and diuretic who contracts a prolonged bout of travellers' diarrhoea. In such a situation there is a greater potential for serious fluid and electrolyte disturbances.

Commonly prescribed drugs in travel medicine and implications for elderly traveller.

Drug–drug interactions where clinically relevant need to be considered, as the elderly are more prone to issues relating to polypharmacye.g. potential contraindications of prescribed travel medicines to conditions more commonly encountered in senior citizens, such as cardiovascular problems and diabetes should also be considered.Seniors are frequently more prone to the adverse effects of drugs,discussed where they are particularly clinically relevant. The points below are not an exhaustive or complete list of all of the prescribing issues, but are presented as an illustration of the principles for careful use of all medicines in the elderly citizens.

*Antimalarials.*It has been reported that some antimalarials lower insulin requirements in diabetic patients and can lead to hypoglycaemia in those treated with insulin or oral hypoglycaemics such as *glibenclamide*. However, the evidence is only available for treatment doses of such antimalarials rather than prophylaxis.There have been limited case reports of an interaction between warfarin and *proguanil and atovaquone/proguanil* resulting in a raised INR. A similar effect has been observed with *doxycycline*. It is wise to monitor the INR of patients taking warfarin after commencing any additional medication such as antimalarials. Also INR should be self monitored for those away longer than 2-3 weeks due to changes in diet and difference in time zones.*Chloroquine* has been reported to cause a rise in digoxin levels in animal models but no clinically important interactions have been observed. Both *chloroquine and mefloquine* also have the potential to increase the risk of arrhythmias if given with other antiarrythmic agents such as amiodarinei.It is best to avoid a range of cardioactive drugs including beta blockers, antiarrythmics and calcium antagonsists in combination with *mefloquine.* This is due to the risk of prolonging the QTc interval and inducing other cardiac adverse effects.Tetracyclines such as *doxyclyine* can have their absorption and therefore efficacy greatly reduced by coadminsitration with antacids based on magnesium, aluminium or carbonate compounds. One ACE inhibitor –quinapril- contains a magnesium carbonate in its formulation sufficient to cause a significant fall in the absorption of teracyclines. *Chloroquine* absorption is also reduced by these antacids.Although caution is recommended when prescribing chloroquine in the presence of renal impairment, no dosage adjustment is necessary in prophylactic use. Tetracyclines such as doxycycline can cause oesophageal damage if not swallowed correctly , sitting upright with ingestion of plenty of water . This could be an issue for those with any swallowing difficulties or prone to oesophageal reflux. There have been reports of increased hypoglycaemia developing in diabetic patients taking glibenclamide when prescribed *ciprofloxacin*, which seems more commonly to occur in the old and In epileptic patients. It is best to avoid *quinolones* for them and also in elderly patients on chronic NSAID treatment due to the risk of convulsions. Tendonitis and tendon rupture have been reported to occur, sometimes within 48 hours of commencing therapy with ciprofloxacin and the risk seems to be greater in those over 60 years of age. It is wise to warn that therapy be discontinued at the first sign of tendon pain, though in most cases, just a single dose is needed to treat Traveller's Diarrhoea.

Azthromycin and others in its class, the macrolides, can cause a rise in digoxin levels, so the combination is best avoided. They should also not be given in combination with other drugs that can prolong that can prolong QT interval.

*Loperamide*The elderly may be more prone to fluid and electrolyte disturbances resulting from a moderate to severe bout of travellers' diarrhoea and the use of oral rehydration therapy is justified. Antidiarrhoeals such as loperamide can also be used as to help control the symptoms though more prolonged therapy may result in constipations.

Analgesic – codeine, tramadol, NSAID   Over the counter narcotic analgesics may also cause constipation and for reasons discussed previously are best avoided when carrying the products across international borders, NSAID induced peptic ulceration is more likely in the elderly as well as the more recently recognised risks of the cardiovascular and renal adverse effects associated with NSAIDs. For occasional use for acute pain, ibuprofen can be carried in the medical kit, but paracetamol is the drug of choice.

Hyoscine containing products for motion sickness are best avoided in the elderly, due to the anticholinergic side effects resulting in potential cardiovascular or other problems, such as urine retention. Hyoscine patches in particular seem to be associated with a high incidence of confusion in the elderly. There is also some evidence of an increased risk of death and mental decline when the over 65s take a combination of drugs with anticholinergic properties, including antihistamines such as chlorpheniramine.

*Proton pump inhibitors (PPIs) and H2 antagonists*This group of medicines are commonly used by older people for self-treatment of dyspeptic symptoms as well as prescribed for peptic ulcer disease. PPIs in particular lower the gastric Ph sufficiently to allow a greater burden of potentially pathogenic organisms to reach the gastrointestinal tract and result in a higher incidence of severe formsof travellers' diarrhoea, a particular problem in the elderly. Those travellers who require continuous PPI therapy might be considered for antibiotic chemoprophylaxis to offer protection against GIT infections.

*Acetazolamide.*Acetazolamide has been associated with a higher risk of metabolic acidosis in the elderly, those with diabetes and in those with reduced renal function. The clearance of acetazolamide is reduced in the presence of a poor renal function resulting in higher blood levels. There is limited data on the occasional use of low dose acetazolamide in the elderly for preventing acute mountain sickness but it should be prescribed with caution in such individuals.It is well doumented that acetazolamide when used in the treatment of glaucoma can produce metabolic acidosis of clinical significance especially in elderly patients and in those with other medical problems. There is also evidence that the elderly have higher blood concentrations of acetazolamide. The BNF recommended dose is 250-1000mg daily, and many patients take a dosage towards the higher end of that range. There is little evidence of the effects of low dose acetazolamide (e.g. 125mg bd as some authorities recommend for the prophylaxis of AMS).In one study of elderly glaucoma patients 75% had blood concentrations increased by a factor of 2, which would equate to a dose of 250mg bd.

Extrapolating this to the use of the drug for AMS, it seems likely that elderly people taking it for AMS are indeed at risk of significant metabolic acidosis. [3-6]

References

1.Baxter K, Stockley's Drug Interactions 9th Edition Pharmaceutical Press, London 2010Sweatman S
2.Martindale (Ed): The complete drug reference 37th Edition. Pharmaceutical Press. London 2011

3. Fukuhara Y, Kaneko T, Orita Y. Nippon Rinsho - Japanese 1992Metabolic acidosis induced by acetazolamide. J. Clinical Medicine. 50 (9):2231-6,
4. Sporn A, Scothorn DM, Terry JE. 1991Acetazolamide blood concentrations are excessive in the elderly.: Propensity for acidosis and relationship to renal function. J .American Optometric Association. 62(12):934-7,
5.Chapron DJ, Gomolin IH, Sweeney KRmetabolic acidosis induced by acetazolamide. Not a rare complication. . J. Clinical Pharmacology. 29(4):348-53, 1989Signifiant
6. Heller I, Halevy J, Cohen S, Theodor E1985 Reply Forward. Archives of Int.Medicine. 145(10):1815-7,

Larry Goodyer

Chapter 12

Travel Health Insurance and Medical Tourism

Preparing for foreign travel

'For my part I travel not to go anywhere, but to go. I travel for travel's sake. The great affair is to move' R L Stevenson.1850

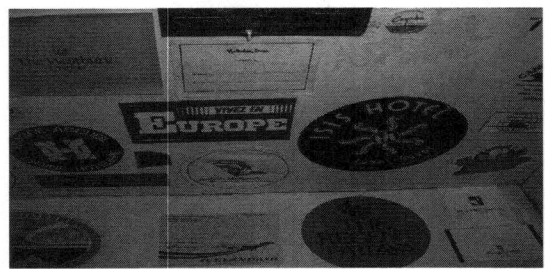

Insuring to ensure good health care abroad.

International translocation without the protection of health insurance protection may threaten the life of the traveller. Many elderly people in ignorance of risk, or cost saving, choose to globe trot without a travel health insurance package. The old and adventurous are at high risk of trauma or ill health while abroad, with cardiac mishap and road traffic accident the most reported health events affecting senior tourists.Many fail to acquire adequate health protection and others purchase inadequate cover, fail to read exclusive small print in the policy, or void it by concealing current infirmity. The number of uninsured or poorly insured older people is likely to increase considerably in future as more insurers refuse to offer policies to older travellers. Many companies have a cut-off age of 65 years, others 70 and few will consider those over 80 years age. Specialist companies still ensure this cohort but the number decreases every year. It is estimated that one in four people go abroad without health insurance cover. Few people arrange cover for trips of less than five days.1

Age Concern calculates that people over 65 years age make 5.5 million trips abroad annually, but they are finding it harder to acquire appropriate travel health insurance protection because of upper age constraints imposed by one in nine insurance providers Three quarters will reject applications for those over 75 years age.1Four out of five insurance claims relate to medical problems and although the old do not have more claims they often cost the insurer more as they are hospitalised more often and for longer.

In the absence of insurance protection medical and nursing care can be prohibitively expensive.e.g.

- A holidaymaker who suffers a heart attack in Greece could face hospital bills of £6,000 to £7,000.
- Repatriation by air ambulance from Spain could cost £10.000
- In the US, treatment for an arm fracture can cost towards£4,000. 000 A serious accident involving an air ambulance can cost £50,000 in the States.Some clinics will only perform operations if they are certain a patient is insured, or can meet the bill. Those without insurance could find themselves with medical bills of ten of thousands of pounds or being refused emergency surgery following injury.Repatriation by air ambulance from Florida to Britain, costs about £30,000 with a similar fee for heart surgery there.
- Hospital costs in popular destinations in France , Greece or Spain embrace ward occupancy rates ranging from £300 daily with medical care to be added. Daily ward rates in USA cost a single day in intensive care up to £10, Some travel health professionals do not perceive it within their role to advise on travel health insurance, but such advice may prove of greater health benefit to the unfortunate ill traveller than recommendations on vaccines and prophylaxis. The adverse impact of a health emergency while the traveller is abroad, especially in developing countries and remote places, may have more dire and immediate consequences than exposure to infection.

Even the best policy will not necessarily provide optimal health care. Provision of service by the travel health insurance industry is dependent upon the quality of resources and health professionals and the evacuation and repatriation possibilities at the venue. Absence, or inadequacy of facilities may defeat the service provider, but the insured is usually assured of the best available care irrespective of cost. The uninsured, at a time of maximal vulnerability, has to cobble together whatever care is attainable often at prohibitive cost, in a situation where geographic, communication and language difficulties are intimidating.

Case History. A 62 man was recently repatriated from southern Greece. He had developed chest pain 17 days previously, was hospitalised, submitted to angiography, followed by triple by-pass surgery and within ten days was ready to return home by air. A similarly aged patient in the next bed had an almost identical history, but was anxiously worrying about future medical care and home return. He had an ECG result which confirmed myocardial infarction but had only been able to have a cardiogram the previous day, which confirmed the need for cardiac surgery. This was too expensive for him to afford and denied access to a flight by the airline, he was contemplating a long road and rail transfer back to the UK, where he would join the long waiting list for surgical intervention. The only difference between the 2 patients was that the first had bought travel health insurance and the second had not purchased any emergency protection. The latter was dependent upon reciprocal EC arrangements, for emergency medical and nursing support and was now facing bills for hospital care. The former had access to the benefits of prompt insurance company attention, immediate medical and surgical intervention and assured speedy repatriation.

The travel health professional, be it nurse, GP or consultant is uniquely placed to offer unbiased advice about insurance protection and should accept the task as part of every pretravel consultation. Attention should be drawn to the need for insurance, contingency evacuation, repatriation, financial reimbursement and the requirement to read the small print, check for exclusions and provide information to insurers of pre-existing illness. Many travel, believing that health protection is in place, but exclusions of which they may be unaware, will have left them unprotected for the conditions most likely to occur while overseas. Others fail to meet contractual obligations to inform the insurer of chronic or existing disorder which abrogates the policy and in emergency they find that cover is not in place or is inadequate.

The travel insurance industry has become more sensitive to higher risk travellers. Elderly travellers may now find that they cannot acquire cover or can only do so at added cost. Annual travel insurance has been largely withdrawn for 90 year plus elders. People who have previously travelled extensively, despite past history of cancer and major cardiac problems, now find themselves with hefty extra premium demands, if they can acquire protection at all. Insurance seekers now face a barrage of questions on life-long health status and current health problems.

The travel health professional should identify the need to advise potential travellers on the hazards of travel without insurance cover. Most travellers are unaware of the inadequacies or expense of health care in developing and affluent countries overseas. They need information on health provision facilities and emergency care, evacuation and repatriation possibilities during their travels, to allow them to make an informed choice about the purchase of insurance cover. They should be encouraged to pay additional premiums for peace of mind and health safety, or be made aware that they travel dangerously if they proceed unprotected.

Policy exclusions often remove activities which thoughtless tourists will undertake while abroad on vacation. Small boat sailing, waterway cruising, paragliding, hill climbing, rafting, small aeroplane and helicopter riding, may all be excluded. Elderly people often appear to cast discretion aside when on vacation and indulge in pursuits they would never contemplate in the home environment. Cover may be absent at the very time when misadventure is most likely to overtake the tourist.

The individual's contractual requirement to advise the insurance company of actual mishap, medical emergency and potential use of services is obligatory, although often a major task when communications between traveller's location and UK may be tenuous.

Case history.A patient died suddenly in Tibet .Direct communication between the British insurer and the involved family could only be established via a fellow traveller's satellite telephone link with the USA through an associated company. Repatriation of the body was beset with difficulties and was only achieved by land transfer via Nepal. Failure to provide the company promptly with a report may negate the contract and expose the patient to substantial costs they cannot meet. It also deprives the support of their expertise and organisation at a time of greatest need.

Elderly global travellers are visiting ever more exotic, developing and remote countries where EHIC and health care reciprocity with the UK does not apply. This fact and insurer resistance to provide cover, higher premiums, rigid adherence to contractual obligations, will mean that more will travel without adequate health protection. In emergency some will find this seriously affects treatment, rehabilitation and repatriation. and they will not receive optimal care in when in urgent need.

All travel health professionals should counsel intending elderly travellers on the benefits of travel health protection and the adequacies of health facilities at their overseas. destination.(See chapter 10) Health professionals are uniquely placed to offer unbiased advice about insurance protection and should accept the task as part of every potential or pretravel consultation. Once clinical fitness for travel has been determined, professional attention should concentrate on insurance cover. Advice should embrace:-

- emergency aid,
- evacuation to hospital,
- quality of care,
- repatriation,
- small print in the insurance policy apropos,
- exclusions to cover,
- terms for pre-existing illness.

Pre-existing conditions and exclusions.

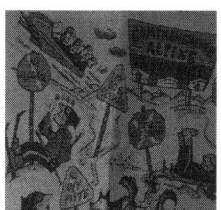

"Pre-existing conditions" can be a catch-all phrase and the opportunity for some companies to refuse claims. However, previously declared medical conditions can be accepted with an extra premium. While most ailments will be insurable, illnesses such as heart disease, or cancer are likely to be excluded from standard policies. Failure to declare any past illness, or one occurring since inception of the policy, may result in rejection of the claim when the insurer contacts the Gp. for personal medical history, on the grounds of failure to meet disclosure requirements. Older holidaymakers are most likely to suffer from disputes about what insurers call "non-disclosure of pre-existing condition" because they are most likely to have suffered relevant illnesses earlier in their lives. The insurer's premise is that they have not had opportunity to assess risk and might have produced a contract with different terms, if they had known about the existing condition. Few people also realise that inebriation at the time of medical mishap may also negate a later insurance claim. 2

Case History An elderly gentleman had a myocardial infarction on a ship cruising off Greenland and had to be helicoptered to hospital in mainland Europe. The bill was expected to be £30,000 and he left behind a disabled wife who had to be disembarked at the first port of call and flown home at additional cost .Insurance covered his care but not his wife's, an expensive oversight.

All travel health professionals should counsel intending travellers on the benefits and weaknesses of travel health protection and the adequacies of overseas health facilities. The Association of British Insurers urges travellers to carry insurance documents at all times, so that doctors treating them will know they are insured. The Foreign Office has warned holidaymakers to be better prepared when taking breaks abroad. They recommend carrying proof of cover on the person, with emergency contact and medical assistance numbers for insurance companies.

Case History. A woman tourist collapsed at the entrance to the Oregon State Legislative building. An on-looker phoned the emergency service and a fire-truck arrived within minutes. The paramedic crew ascertained she was still living, their second check was to seek and find her insurance document. This was perused. She was promptly placed on a trolley and sped off to a private unit, examined and warded within an hour. In its absence she would have been taken to the local state hospital with a very lengthy wait for attention with admission problematic.

Older people should consider travel insurance as a necessity not an option. The travel insurance industry has however toughened its approach to at risk travellers, particularly older travellers and the very elderly. This process may now require considerable endeavour and for some this is a disincentive to act. Elderly travellers may now find that they cannot find cover or can only do so at considerable added cost. Annual cover has been largely withdrawn for the very old. Patients, who have travelled extensively despite a past clinical history, now face premium loading, if they can acquire protection at all.

The number of insurers catering for elderly people has fallen dramatically. On line search a year ago would have provided many sources but few are now displayed and they prove selective. Potential insurance buyers must answer many questions on life-long health status and current health problems, and may be excluded on initial screening. Any inaccuracy in disclosure at this time, or once the cover is in place, may void a later claim. Those having difficulties in acquiring cover should insist on by-passing the initial screener and accessing the insurer's clinical appraiser who may have a more realistic stance and be prepared to take on the risk.

Travel health insurance doesn't cover every eventuality but only closely defined levels of risk. As insurance premiums have fallen in a competitive market, insurers now adhere to policy wording. For example, pre-existing medical conditions of relatives are common exclusions in travel policies. The death of a close relative from a pre-existing medical condition would not be covered under the terms and conditions of many policies, if the condition was known to the customer prior to the commencement of the period of insurance. There is usually no cover in place for cancelling or curtailing a holiday on account of a relative's illness or death if the relative has a terminal condition, or has been to a hospital (including outpatient consultations), or has taken prescribed medication within 90 days of departure date. Holidaymakers should also remember that if they want to travel for more than 45 days they must always confirm with their insurer before assuming they are covered.

Case History. A patient returned from a holiday in Morocco having paid a considerable medical care bill when he developed severe chest pain for which he was hospitalised. He believed his health insurance company would foot the bill but the small print specifically excluded ill health of cardiac cause after he had suffered a previous coronary artery .He had failed to read the insurance document before the premium was paid –an expensive mistake not uncommonly made by members of the travelling public

Insurance Provision

The cost of annual worldwide, multi-trip travel insurance for a couple over the age of 75 can range from £184 from "insurefor.com "to £325 from the online provider" getmy.com. A new service offered to M&S credit card holders provides annual worldwide, multi-trip travel insurance for couples up to the age of 80 for £120 a year and includes travel to the US, Canada and the Caribbean. The small print of the M&S reveals comprehensive levels of cover, with £10m medical expenses and £2m personal liability cover included.

A British insurance company has claimed to be the first to offer cover against Deep-Vein Thrombosis (DVT).P J Hayman, an online insurance provider offers emergency medical assistance cover for travellers contracting DVT and £10,000 should death occur during the trip or within 72 hours of the policyholder's arriving home. Most cheap policies exclude all claims – even medical claims- made as a result of: war, invasion, acts of foreign enemies, hostilities or warlike operations (whether war be declared or not), civil war, rebellion, terrorism, revolution, insurrection, civil commotion made in connection with those countries to which the Foreign Office has advised people to avoid "all but essential travel".

Summary

Elderly travellers are visiting more exotic, developing and remote countries where EHIC protection does not apply.

People are booking flights and accommodation separately on line (50% of holidays) by-passing the travel agent and making it more likely that many will travel uninsured.

Insurer resistance to provide cover, higher premiums, rigid adherence to contractual obligations, mean that more will travel without adequate health protection. In emergency this will seriously affect treatment, rehabilitation and repatriation.

All travel health professionals should counsel intending travellers on the benefits of travel health protection and the adequacies or deficiencies of health facilities at overseas destinations.

Health Insurance and Repatriation

Travel insurance like household insurance involves underwriters, brokers, claim handlers, customer services and y the potential patient. To help process claims travel insurers have a medical unit. Manned 24 hours, 365 days a week by doctors, nurses and support staff these deal with the first calls, follow up with local doctor and hospital on a regular basis, confirm a diagnosis and contact a UK GP to ensure that the individual had no relevant undeclared previous medical history. If insurance cover is provided the medical desk assesses the need for medical care. It deals with issues such as the transfer of the client to better hospital care, and repatriation to the UK. Repatriation can be non-air (road ambulance from France), scheduled, charter air craft seats in Europe),or true air ambulance. Costs vary from several thousand to a million pounds.

An escort may be required – a non-medical person/doctor/nurse as a team or individual. The accompanying doctor will travel with patient from foreign to home bedside .The medical team will be appropriately equipped by the insurer with defibrillators or ventilators as required. Transport is arranged to meet the aeroplane and the patient safely transferred to a pre-arranged hospital. At the point of handover to an NHS, private facility or home the responsibilities of the insurance medical team cease.

Criteria for repatriation include: genuine medical necessity, poor local facilities, difficult access, cost and patient preference (where this is deemed by the insurer to be reasonable).

People who rely on the protection afforded by possession of the EHIC are often unaware that it does not cover repatriation, or medical/nursing care for the return to UK.,

Exclusions from insurance cover are common. They vary significantly between policies. The following are examples: No cover is provided if:-

- taking continuing medication
- have had medical treatment or surgery within the last 6 months
- are suffering from a previously diagnosed psychiatric disorder
- have any AIDS related complex

Exclusions are sometimes vague and it is vital to :-

- read the insurance small print
- declare past medical history
- get expert travel medical advice

Consideration: Careful thought should be given to travel location and quality of local facilities for those with pre-existing illness.

Those with breathlessness on the ground should seek expert advice before being exposed to air flight which, despite pressurisation, is equivalent to a height of about 2,500 m..

Insurers will pay what they think they need to pay – an air-ambulance will not be sent out for a trivial claim and they may insist on land as opposed to air transfer, a nurse rather than a medical escort. Repatriation arrangements often take place with patient and supporting relative in a vulnerable negotiating situation.

EC Health Protection

The European Health Insurance Card (or EHIC) allows anyone who is insured by, or covered by a statutory social security scheme of the EEA countries and Switzerland to receive medical treatment in another member state for free or at a reduced cost, if that treatment becomes necessary during their visit (for example, due to illness or an accident), or if they have a chronic pre-existing condition which requires care such as kidney dialysis. The intention of the scheme is to allow people to continue their stay in a country without having to return home for medical care; as such, it does not cover people who have visited a country for the purpose of obtaining medical care, nor does it cover care, such as many types of dental treatment, which can be delayed until the visitor returns home. It only covers healthcare which is normally covered by a statutory health care system in the visited country, so it does not render travel insurance unnecessary. Many travellers still fail to organise EC reciprocal health protection, or are unaware that it requires regular renewal.[4]

The EHIC has limitations. Quality of care depends upon national provision, which may be of poorer quality and resource than that provided by the NHS. It does not provide for repatriation. It does not guarantee full financial recompense for medical and hospital bills and does not cover transportation to a hospital. Private health insurance is still advisable in time of need if only for repatriation cover.* A certificate of entitlement by application through a post office, or on-line -is required for cover to be obtained, a minor inconvenience in return for considerable emergency health support in EC countries. This protection should not be spurned and many insurance companies will only provide cover if the insured has utilised EC cover in emergency. Change to EC regulations means that former certificates are no longer valid. New ones need to be acquired and renewed every three years. Britons still travel without basic EHIC protection. Travellers should be aware that some common tourist destinations such as Turkey and north Cyprus are not within the EC and therefore EHIC does not apply.

The card is applicable in all French overseas departments (Martinique, Guadeloupe, Réunion and French Guiana) as they are part of the EEA, but not non-EEA dependent territories such as Jersey, Isle of Man, Aruba or French Polynesia. However there are agreements for the use of the EHIC in the Faroe Islands ,Greenland even though they are not in the EEA.and Switzerland is also included.(www.ehic/ie)

Recommendations

Health professional should consider it a duty to advise potential travellers on the hazards of travel without insurance cover and recommend acquisition of EHIC protection.

Elderly Travellers should be made aware of the inadequacies and expense of health care in overseas countries to be visited. They should be advised to acquire information on health provision facilities, emergency care and evacuation and repatriation possibilities during travel, to permit informed choice. They travel dangerously if proceeding without insurance protection

Individuals should be reminded of contractual requirements to advise the insurance company immediately of mishap, medical emergency and potential use of services even when communications between the travellers location and UK may be tenuous. Failure to provide the company promptly with a report may negate the contract and deprive them of support and expertise in time of need. Failure to utilise EHIC may void the insurance claim.

Summary

- Older travellers should acquire EHIC protection and be aware of its limitations.
- Elderly travellers are visiting more exotic, developing and remote countries where EC reciprocal Health Protection does not apply.
- DIY holiday arrangements, with many booking flights and accommodation separately on line by-passing the travel agent, make it more likely that many will travel uninsured.
- Insurer resistance to provide cover, higher premiums, rigid adherence to contractual obligations, mean that more old people will travel without adequate health protection. In emergency this will seriously affect treatment, rehabilitation and repatriation.

Medical tourism

Medical tourism-*travel with the prime intent of seeking investigation, treatment and operative intervention abroad*-is a growing industry in several countries in the developing world. Affluent older people with failing systems and disabilities are attracted to medical tourism as it presents an opportunity to travel and save money. Nearly 450,000 foreigners sought medical treatment in India in 2007 with Singapore not far behind and Thailand in the lead with over a million medical tourists. One in twenty people interviewed recently have had a medical or dental procedure out with the UK, or are planning one. [5]

The British Medical Association has stated that thorough research is essential on quality of care and resources before a person should consider going abroad for treatment. Patients should investigate all aspects of the proposed treatment. This must include the health and safety standards of facilities and the potential impact of long distance travel on the recovery from medication or surgery received while abroad. People with pre-existing illness should therefore satisfy themselves that adequate facilities for treatment will be available if complications arise and whether the risk is justified of being outwith the NHS umbrella of post treatment care.

No global regulatory body exists to appraise quality of care provided in overseas institutions engaged in medical tourism. There is a universal body for accreditation, the International

Society for Quality in Health Care (ISQua), which has members in 70 countries. Medtral New Zealand also caters for people looking for more affordable treatment abroad. The Joint Commission International (JCI) accredits hospitals, while QHA Trent, a British company, accredits and provides consultancy services for hospitals and clinics globally.

Potentials patients should check the surgeon's training, patient testimonials and published " adverse events" and if they are independently verified. Some hospitals refer to overall adverse event rate. If they do thousands of eye operations and endoscopies their adverse event rate is very low compared to a unit doing complex major surgery. Checks need also to made on the level of English spoken and after-care facilities One survey found that 43% of British patients travelled abroad for dental treatment, 29% for cosmetic surgery and the remainder for orthopaedic and infertility surgery.5.6

In 2009 more than 50,000 Britons went abroad for surgery; In 2011 the number is expected to be at least 75,000, according to Treatmentabroad.net, a website for medical tourists. The company provides information on hospitals, clinics and specialists worldwide. Among the more popular treatments are cosmetic surgery and dentistry, which are expensive in the UK and often may not be covered by private insurance. The cost of a cheap flight, plus the cost of surgery along with a few days of rest and recuperation, may be much cheaper than having the work done at home. Booking through an agent permits negotiation of an all-inclusive package and patients are likely to get better before, during and after care.

Travellers are really having surgery as part of a holiday or business trip. It is possible, for instance, to combine cosmetic surgery or dental treatment with a safari in South Africa, and a hip replacement or knee surgery with a trip to Thailand or India. An inclusive check-up provided by BUPA in UK. may cost £430 and a similar well person health check at a Hospital in Bangalore, including chest x-rays, full torso ultrasound, lung function test, electrocardiogram and a battery of other blood, urine and diagnostic tests, may cost just £23. Included in the price is a consultation with a doctor to discuss any worrying findings and recommendations on health improvements. The patient is given x-rays, printouts and reports to show the GP at home. Patients should be aware however that consultants overseas will not have access to previous investigations and clinical notes available to the individual when being treated within the NHS at home. This lack of global knowledge of the patient's past clinical exposure may be disadvantageous if the patient has a complex history and chronic illness.

The Foreign & Commonwealth Office warns *that, although medical and dental treatment abroad may be cheaper, "standards of care in some countries may not be the same as those in the UK, and emergency facilities such as intensive care may not be readily available"*. In some countries, there may be a risk of transmission of blood viruses such as HIV, hepatitis B and hepatitis C during medical procedures. Tattoos and body piercing should be avoided in overseas situations because of the risk of infection.

People mistakenly believe that travel insurance policies will cover elective surgery abroad, just because they cover an accidental occurrence that leads to them requiring medical treatment. Conventional policies and the EHIC will not provide cover for medical costs if the individual has elected to travel abroad for care. Specialist " enhanced medical " insurance policies are available at an appropriate premium.

Countries involved in Medical Tourism

Bulgaria. Some private clinics are now highly regarded in Bulgaria and Northern Europeans increasingly choose Bulgaria for 'Hospital Vacations' - receiving treatment at a very reasonable cost compared to Western Europe, followed by recuperation in one of Bulgaria's famous spas. Healing waters at Hissar, and Bankya, are thought to bring relief to arthritis and rheumatism sufferers.

Croatia .Medical Tourism facilities are well established and often incorporate traditional spa and hydrotherapy

Thailand. The Kasikorn Research Centre reported that 1.28 million expatriates visited Thai Hospitals in 2005, generating considerable revenue .Procedures were major surgery, out patient clinic visits ,annual check-ups. Bumrungrad Hospital treated 400,000 foreign patients in 2005 .The hospital has a new 18-story outpatient centre, Bangkok Hospital, with affiliated hospitals (like BNH Hospital, Samitivej Hospital and branches in Pattaya and Phuket) is also a popular destination for medical tourists. Standard of treatment and technology can be high with prices lower than in other countries providing similar quality and technology. Thailand is developing as a medical hub for patients from the United States, Europe, Far and Middle East

India

Medical tourism in India has been growing recently and is a popular destination for medical tourists who receive effective medical treatment at lower costs than in developed countries. India's medical tourism sector is expected to experience an annual growth rate of 30%,. Estimates of the value of medical tourism to India go as high as $2 billion a year by 2012.As medical treatment costs in the developed world surge upwards Westerners consider international travel for medical care increasingly appealing. 150,000 people travel to India for low-priced health care procedures every year. The advantages for medical tourists include reduced costs, availability of latest medical technologies and a growing compliance on international quality standards. Britons are less likely to face a language barrier in India.

Estimates claim treatment costs in India start at around a tenth of the price of comparable treatment in Britain. Popular Indian treatments are alternative medicine, bone-marrow transplant, cardiac bypass, eye surgery and hip replacement. India is known in particular for heart surgery, hip resurfacing and other areas of advanced medicine. The south Indian city of Chennai nets in 45% of health tourists. Some hospitals in Chennai are equipped with state of the art medical equipment and costs are relatively inexpensive city compared to Mumbai

(Bombay) and Delhi. The Indian medical tourist healthcare delivery system is striving to match international standards. 13 Indian hospitals have been accredited by the Joint Commission International (JCI) acknowledging standardized protocols and safety.

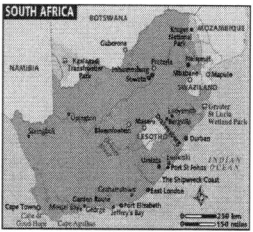

South Africa.

Standards in South African clinics are on a par with UK clinics. Prices and quality of care vary across the country. Patients travelling to South Africa should check their surgeons' qualifications are genuine before treatment. The most popular treatment is cosmetic surgery but the country also provides organ transplants, heart, orthopaedic and obesity surgery and dentistry.

Surgeons training in South Africa undertake an extensive 12 year training programme before they qualify. Most surgeons study in the US or the UK before providing care in South Africa.

Patients can expect to save 40 – 60% on treatment compared with UK. Hospitals and clinics in South Africa are vying to attract more international medical tourism patients from around the world. Although the cost of medical treatment is not as price competitive as other popular medical travel destinations, the quality of treatment is very good.

Singapore:

As a leading healthcare services hub in Asia, Singapore attracts 200,000 international patients every year.. Many international patients place their confidence in Singapore's world class healthcare system, which is at the forefront of medical technology and has safety as top priority The Singapore Government aims to attract close to a million overseas patients by the year 2012. Singapore competes with Thailand and Malaysia to grab a slice out of the medical tourism cake.

Malaysia

Malaysia is among the world's top five medical tourism destinations for medical tourists selected on quality and affordability of medical care. It ranks third behind Panama and Brazil, and followed by Costa Rica and India., Malaysia's medical tourism industry has seen considerable growth in recent years. From 2001 to 2006, the number of foreigners seeking healthcare services in Malaysia almost tripled from 75,210 patients to 296,687 patients. Much of Malaysia's attraction lies in the wide array of medical services and procedures including dental, cosmetic and cardiac surgeries at significantly lower costs compared with Europe. 35 private hospitals in the country have been identified to promote Malaysia as a health tourist destination. Malaysia's growing reputation on the world healthcare map has also been recognised by a number of international and regional medical associations.

Ukraine. The Crimea coast of Ukraine has a long history of spa therapy and is now endeavouring to attract medical tourists from Europe. Standards of care vary with the institution.

Personal Health Protection

- Older travellers should acknowledge individual responsibility for personal health maintenance while overseas and insure themselves against mishap in pretravel and en route preparation. They should:-
- Acquire appropriate vaccinations and prophylaxis.
- Use mechanical means of protection against malaria eg repellents.
- Take measures to avoid infected food and water.
- Acquaint themselves with health hazards en route and at destination
- Be aware of emergency health care facilities at destination
- Carry a list of medications
- Carry on the person at all times routine medications
- Recognise the limitations of travel health insurance and EHIC protection
- Acknowledge that increasing age makes them higher health risk travellers.

References

1. McIntosh I Travel health Insurance , 2007 Brit. Trav. Health Assoc. J.10.58-59
2 McIntosh I Adequate Travel Insurance , 2004 Brit. Trav. Health Assoc. J 5. 41-42
3 McIntosh I EHIC insurance . 2010 In the News Brit. Trav. Health Assoc. J .15.69-60
4 McIntosh I Insurance ,in the news.2011 Brit. Trav. Health Assoc. J .16.37
5 McIntosh I Medical Tourism in the news.2011 Brit. Trav. Health Assoc. J 1637-8
6 Fairhurst R. in Travellers |Health ed. Dawood R. Oxford Univ, Press 2002

Insurers catering for older travellers

Among the companies that offer full cover are Direct Travel Insurance (0845 605 2500, www.direct-travel.co.uk: from £48 for an annual policy/£24 for a 17-day single trip); Norwich Union Direct (0808 101 6705, www.norwichunion.com), and members of the British Insurance Brokers Association (0870 950 1790, www,biba.org.uk).

Useful websites

www. Insuresupermarket.com
www.medictravel.com
www.insureandgo.com
www.flexicover.com.
www.ehic/ie

Iain B. McIntosh

Chapter 13

Emergency Health Care while Abroad.

Many older people travel the world believing that holiday health insurance will ensure optimal quality emergency evacuation, medical care and repatriation. It may, but much depends upon local facilities at location of injury, or illness. Quality and availability of resources vary markedly between regions, countries and localities. Climatic season and transportation infrastructure also affect evacuation and repatriation. Older people are more likely than the young to become ill while abroad, are likely to be hospitalised for longer and require medical repatriation.[1]. Elderly tourists should be aware of the quality of health resources they may meet in time of need. They should investigate and consider the quality of service, speed of response and ease of repatriation when planning their holiday. Travel health professionals should draw attention to these preparations in pretravel clinic consultations.

Emergency Health Care

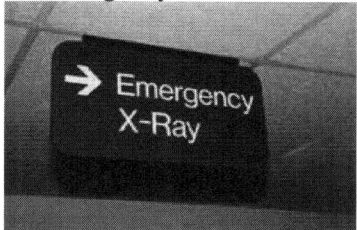

Emergency Health Care Abroad can be categorised for quality of care and the following tourist destinations are considered:-

North and Western Europe
Eastern Europe and Danube cruises
The Mediterranean coastlands
Baltic and Black sea Cruising
Caribbean Islands
Middle East
North America
South America
West Africa and African safaris
Asia and Far East
Australia New Zealand
Extreme Latitudes

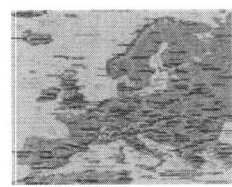

Emergency Health Care Within Europe

Many tourists travel within and along the coasts of Europe and ill Britons can now often obtain speedy, high quality care in countries within the European Union. The EHIC card covers emergency health care in the 27 members of the EC and a few other states. Standard of resources and medical care however varies within European boundaries. Britons using this service must present a EHIC card entitling them to free medical treatment within the European Economic area. Insurance organisations may not reimburse treatment claims if it has not been produced at the point of treatment.2 The member countries of the European Union (2011) are:

Austria, Belgium, Bulgaria, Cyprus, Czech Republic, Denmark, Estonia, Finland, France, Germany, Greece, Hungary, Ireland, Italy, Latvia, Lithuania, Luxembourg, Malta, Netherlands, Poland, Portugal, Romania, Slovakia, Slovenia, Spain, Sweden, United Kingdom and reciprocation includes Canary Islands, Azores, Madeira and French Guyana, Guadeloupe, Martinique. The European Health Insurance Card (EHIC) allows individual access to state-provided healthcare in all European Economic Area (EEA) countries and Switzerland at a reduced cost, or sometimes, free of charge. Applying for the card is free and it is valid for five years. Presenting the EHIC CARD entitles the bearer to treatment necessary during the trip, but does not allow travel abroad specifically to receive medical care. However, renal dialysis and management of pre-existing or, chronic, conditions that arise while abroad are all covered by the EHIC. It allows access to the same state-provided healthcare as a resident of the country being visited. However, many of thee countries expect the patient to pay towards cost of treatment.

France. Linked closely by rail and sea to the UK, is the country most visited by Britons. There is no great difference in quality of care between private and public hospitals in France and little difference in price. Treatment, whether private or public, is not free at point of delivery. Patients pay the full bill and are then reimbursed later. Being treated in private clinics in France does not mean avoiding waiting lists as they do not exist, but going private does not mean footing the entire bill .3.

Germany. East German general practice under communism was tightly controlled in large polyclinics. City doctors are now encouraged to run single handed practices as in West Germany. Visitors pay the Gp. and claim a refund if they have produced an EHIC card. In **Germany, Poland Slovenia, Hungary, Slovakia, Austria, Czech Republic, Spain, Portugal and Italy** GPs usually work single handed ,are unlikely to have practice nurses and do not practice gynaecology. Health centres in Spain and Portugal employ salaried doctors.Home visits are infrequent, with out of hours work done by co-operatives working out of hospitals, or health centres. In France, Spain and Germany, it is now advantageous for travellers who suffer acute cardiac problems to undertake immediate by-pass surgery abroad, rather than return to the UK to be wait listed.4

Spain. A network of private and state health institutions and EC reciprocal health care ensure Britons can expect as good and often better health care in emergency than in the UK. Travel health insurance companies now organise clients requiring cardiac intervention, stent insertion and by-pass surgery to receive this in Spain for prompt efficient service. In Spanish hospitals along the tourist dominated Mediterranean coast, there are dedicated English translators on call to ease linguistic problems.

Italy. The country ranks second on the WHO list of countries for top quality health care services. However, many public hospitals are overcrowded and underfunded, although medical facilities are adequate for emergencies. Visitors are expected to pay full hospital charges and then claim reimbursement from their insurance provider. In case of emergency, most general and regional hospitals have emergency rooms (pronto soccorso), open 24 hours a day.

Greece. Greece's public health system provides free or low cost health care for those who contribute to Greek social security. Although medical training is of a high standard, the health service is one of the worst in Europe, largely because of under-funding. Public hospitals are inundated with patients. Standards of hygiene are high however and hospital virus infection almost non-existent. In Greece GPs are replaced by internists, who are physicians doing primary care work. A large hospital on Corfu, a favoured tourist island, has recently been completed. In some hospitals patient eating resources have to be provided by relatives, which present a problem for an ill unaccompanied tourist. Hospital and A&E departments are often manned by private doctors.

Malta and Cyprus. In Malta and Cyprus, favoured holiday spots for Britons of retiral age, most GPs work privately. A large central regional hospital has been completed recently in Malta. In the Maltese state and private sector, diabetes is managed in secondary care and GPs may not even arrange x-rays to check for fractures. In Cypriot and Greek towns, hospital and A&E departments are manned by private doctors.

Landfall on European river cruises

British tourists visit the European community on land tours and transit many countries in east and west Europe on river cruises. Small ships, without on-board doctors, cruise along the rivers Danube and Rhine and are popular with aging and often ailing tourists. They are reassured by the thought that reciprocal health arrangements will provide for emergency health care. The majority of countries neighbouring the Danube in its long course are members of the EC, with a few exceptions such as Serbia and Croatia and Albania. The standard of available emergency medical care and facilities varies greatly, with cross border travel.(5)

In Western Europe, high quality resources equate with those in the NHS and are immediately available. In eastern European countries, struggling health care systems may not provide the urgent care the ill traveller requires. Immediacy of assistance may also be a problem, as rivers run through many rural areas far from population centres, where ambulance transfer may be unavailable. Private health insurers therefore may not be able logistically, to provide optimal care for tourists in emergency. Insurance companies can only provide what is available from local resources and the patient may have to augment financial agreements, with "informal arrangements"-bribes. (6)

Romania This is a poor Balkan country and new European Community. It is shedding a culture of Communist corruption, when bribery affected every administrative system, including health care. Medical care in Romania is generally not up to Western standards, and basic medical supplies are limited, especially outside major cities .The country's health care system is so underfinanced, that it faces imminent collapse. Even large university hospitals often lack surgical gloves, antibiotics and medication, forcing patients to pay for them. Buildings are in need of repair with rusting surgical instruments, dilapidated examination beds, cracked, damp walls and dirty toilets common. Private medical providers meeting Western quality standards are available in Bucharest and other cities but can be difficult to locate.

Doctors are still accustomed to receiving bribes and low average monthly medical wages encourage bribe-taking. Patients pay more to get good clinical and nursing attention.6Transparency International, ranked Romania as the second most corrupt country in the 27-member European Union in 2010, behind Bulgaria. A World Bank report concluded that "informal payments" amounted to £200 million annually. Ethically practising doctors observe that the bribery culture is so established that, when bribes are refused ,patients mistakenly believe it a sign that illnesses are incurable! Bribery will be required from the ill tourist and costs range from £75 for appendicectomy to £4000 for surgery, with prices posted on blogs and Web sites.

Considerations

- Potential health risks within Romania include hepatitis A, polio, typhoid, and rabies – Travellers to Romania should ensure they are up to date on all routine and hepatitis immunizations. Dental treatment, tattoos and injections should be avoided when within the country and its neighbours.

- Travellers seeking medical treatment should choose provider carefully as quality care is scarce and endeavour to get treatment at a well-equipped centre by travelling to county or capital hospital, where staff may speak English. Visitors must tip medical personnel to guarantee that sufficient attention is given to their medical conditions.

Hungary. Hungary transformed its healthcare system to a decentralised model and now has EC reciprocity. All citizens are covered, regardless of employment status, Patients make co-payments on certain services, including pharmaceuticals and dental car(7GPs contract with the Hungarian Insurance Fund and provide a prescription and referral service 8. In hospitals, the fee-for-service payment scheme encourages hospitals to treat for financial gain.9. The system often sees doctors doing nursing duties. (3). Apart from out-of-pocket payments for pharmaceuticals and dental care, 'gratitude 'payments-bribes- by patients, continue to play an important role

Consideration. Unaware tourists unprepared to offer bribes will receive inferior care. 10

Bulgaria. The Bulgarian healthcare system is slowly catching up with Western European nations. Citizens have access to a free national health service. Medical equipment in many establishments is in poor condition, often more than 20 years old and the health care system is in a critical state. Medical staff are trained to high standard, receive low wages and operate inadequate and outdated machinery. Hospitals and clinics may not have the equipment and facilities expected in Western Europe. Dentists work privately and pharmacists offer affordable, unregulated treatment and medicines. Transparency International, ranked Bulgaria the most corrupt country in the European Union in 2010. There are a growing number of private hospitals and clinics and state clinics and medical services in all major towns and cities. Nursing care can be sparse, and knowledge of English limited. 11

Consideration.

- Doctors and hospitals may expect immediate payment in cash for health services. "Informal and gratitude "payments are often expected for simple medical and nursing attention.

- Dental treatment, tattoos and injections should be avoided if possible when within the country.

- Visitors should purchase comprehensive private travel medical insurance which should include medical evacuation to Britain.

Serbia. Serbia has weathered years of political and economic turmoil, ethnic strife and civil war. The country has a well developed network of primary/secondary care centres, but the system is inefficient and underfunded with equipment and facilities out of date, staff underpaid and demoralised. A European Agency study found that only a third of hospitals had functioning sterilisation equipment and 75% of the medical equipment in health facilities was more than 10 years old. Conditions are improving but vary across the country and medical care is limited. Physicians in Serbia are well-trained, but hospitals and clinics lack equipment and supplies and in large parts of rural Serbia, ambulance service may be unavailable. In acute emergency, best option is Military Medical Academy Belgrade.12

Consideration.

- Health workers routinely accept" on the side" informal payments from patients and supplement income with private practice. Patients have to buy hospital supplies "out-of-pocket", even for items such as bandages and catheters.

- Venous injections and acupuncture should be avoided if possible when within the country.

Croatia.Large parts of the country were devastated by recent war and medical facilities vary widely across the region, with best resources along the Dalmatian coast. Here Medical Tourism facilities are well established. Privatisation of primary health care (except for emergency and public health services) is under way, with about one third of primary care doctors specialists in general medicine, General practitioner-led primary health care is central to the newly organised health care system. Patients have a free choice of primary care doctor the gatekeeper to secondary care in polyclinic or hospital. Those in work and their families have access to state health care, which is covered by government-subsidized medical insurance. Over-all, facilities are good with free emergency aid available for the tourist in emergency. Major population centres have decent private health care facilities. Zagreb is best served with a large general hospital 13

Albania. Healthcare in Albania is mainly public/state and only partly private. The rural population and especially those in the north-eastern part of the country have lower standard of living and of healthcare than elsewhere. There are plans to privatise parts of the healthcare system, to improve existing infrastructure and to build new institutions. Currently there are shortages of medicines, medical equipment and hospitals are dilapidated. The qualifications of medical personnel have not been carefully regulated and nurses and doctors can still expect "informal payments " to ensure patient attention.300 healthcare centres have been refurbished and some hospitals and polyclinics in cities have also been renovated and some modern diagnostic and treatment equipment installed. Assistance from the European Community has distributed medical equipment to 500 healthcare centres and 2200 clinics and there has been privatisation of pharmacies. A few private facilities are available to tourists in Tirana but quality of care for the ill elderly tourist away from the capital is problematic with emergency transportation a further difficulty.

Consideration. Health care and resources vary markedly across the country and emergency

aid may be delayed.

- Dental treatment, tattoos and injections should be avoided when within the country. Travellers seeking medical treatment should choose provider carefully as quality care is scarce
- Tourists must tip medical personnel to guarantee that sufficient attention is given to medical conditions

Switzerland Although not a member of the EU, the country has reciprocal arrangements and the EHIC card can be used in emergency giving access to good facilities.

Summary

Medical and nursing care resources and facilities vary greatly in countries bordering the Rivers Danube and Rhine, particularly in the Balkans. The river based tourist may meet care as good as, or better than, within the NS, or be exposed to conditions closer to those met in an undeveloped country of the third world. Cruise ships without crew doctor or nurse, pass through many rural areas where health care is limited and falls far short of that available in the big cities. Tourists should remember that they cannot wholly escape the use of local health care resources in emergency. Private health insurance can only provide the best that is available locally and repatriation may be tenuous and lengthy. The public healthcare systems in Central and Eastern Europe have often been declining during the past decade and are underfunded, lack solid infrastructure and are unable to keep professional medical staff in the country.

Round the Mediterranean

Elderly vacationers now holiday and reside for part of the year in large number along the Mediterranean littoral, the Adriatic and on many of their islands. Many of the countries along the shores are within the European Community and offer good and relatively standardised health care to travellers who become ill or are injured.

In developing regions and those out-with the EC bloc, standards vary and can be very poor. Tourists often only become aware of inadequacies in health facilities and support when overtaken by a medical or traumatic crisis and can suffer from delayed, or poor, intervention in emergency. Chance can also determine whether the patient under duress is exposed to state established or private health care. The response to an emergency may be delivered by a private or state sponsored ambulance, which will decant the patient into the respective health care sector, with each providing very different standards of provision and support. Linguistic difficulties and cultural differences can also create problems for those in medical need.

In general, the developed countries of the region operate private and state funded medical care, with tourists protected by travel health insurance benefiting from exposure to the former. EC reciprocity ensures that the uninsured will receive emergency care equivalent to that of the countries citizens. The EHIC card does not cover the cost of repatriation. Away from mainland Italy, France and Spain however private health care may predominate and place the uninsured at risk from an inadequacy or absence of care for foreign visitors. 14

Spain.Italy.France. Portugal. British visitors are assured of good health support along the coastal fringe. Reciprocity ensures access to health care for all UK residents in emergency. Private care predominates in the south of Italy and in Adriatic resorts. There are many English-speaking and foreign doctors in resort areas and major cities. In Portugal nursing care and post-hospital assistance are below what most northern Europeans anticipate

Morocco, Algeria.Tunisia. Libya and Egypt. There may be scant or absent universal health care for citizenry and private health care predominates. State institutions may be embryonic, inadequate and offer services far below standards across the sea. Quality of resources deteriorates with distance from major population centres and may be rudimentary in the rural scene. Tourists can expect good private facilities in major cities and some emergency state provision, but in developing townships rural and small and new tourist venues, good care may be distant. Immediate first aid and casualty evacuation facilities may not exist. 15 The recent revolutions in Tunisia and Egypt bring even more uncertainty to availability of health care within the country and the war in Libya has ravaged itshealth care system.

Morocco. The country has inadequate numbers of physicians and hospital beds and poor access to water and sanitation. The health care system includes 122 hospitals, 2,400 health centres, which are poorly maintained and lack adequate capacity to meet demand for medical care. Tourists located far from major centres and venturing into the hinterland should be aware there are few immediate response vehicles, and access to any good hospital may be hours away. Travel health insurance can only provide what is available and local provision may be non-existent, with transfer to a unit with good facilities some time away. In emergency, road traffic accident and bodily trauma exposes the traveller to admission to local facilities, where hygiene standards may be questionable.

Consideration.

- People travelling without travel health insurance cover may expect a modicum of emergency provision, but ambulance transfer, medication and surgical intervention must be paid for as well as the hotel element of hospitalisation.

- Emergency fluid and blood transfusion brings risks from contamination, HIV infection and hepatitis

Algeria. In Algeria a system of almost free national health care exists. Hospitalisation, medicines, and outpatient care are free to all. Most health services are provided by the public sector, although a small private sector has been expanding.

Libya. Before the war Libya with its remarkable Roman antiquities was opening up to tourism. Tripoli and Benghazi offered good private health care with some free health provision for the general populace. There was a medium quality health care system, accessible for all citizens, but affected by the international trade embargo, with import of equipment and medicines difficult.A network of small hospitals serve the littoral areas of Tripolitania and Cyrenaica. Health units with basic facilities exist in Derna and Tobruk which before the war were being visited by cruise ships and tourists touring the antiquities. These were small units with limited facilities. The revolution of the populace has had adverse effects on the universality of health care in the country increasing variation in quality of care between east and west, rural and city parts of the country.

Egypt. Holiday resorts extend from El Alamein to Alexandria along the Mediterranean and up the River Nile. A good transport system brings within reach, Cairo and Alexandria and prime hospital facilities in state and private sector. Public hospitals are open to tourists. Standard of care is good in Cairo and Alexandria but varies in other parts of the country. Health care provision is lacking in remote rural areas, particularly in Western Desert oases. The 2011 revolution brings uncertainty to the health care scene.

Israel. The Health care system is reputed to be one of the most advanced in the world. The State has maintains a system of socialized health care. Providers in the Israeli system consist of a mixture of private, semi-private and public entities. Cruise ships calling at Haifa can off load ill patients and expect good local and centralised care.

Syria. has a well-developed health care system in the cities, involving state and private hospitals, many public and private outpatient clinics and different sorts of health centres. The health system for the rural areas is limited with few services and the country has problems with tuberculosis infection.

Turkey. has a very complex health care system of variable quality, especially in most state hospitals. Private hospitals have raised the quality of their physicians and medical equipment. Most hospitals and doctors are concentrated in cities and big towns. Private health insurance is well developed in major centres and most popular tourist resorts. A scant health service exists in rural areas with large distances between emergency aid locations and poor transportation facilities in the hinterland.

Albania. has a health care system in transition. It offers basic primary health care system, but many facilities were damaged in conflict up to 1997 and deficits are present in expertise, skills and management. Facilities remain publicly owned with the exception of licensed private pharmacies and dentists.(See chap.12 on European River Cruises.)

Croatia.Greece See chap. 12on EC countries).

Summary.

When travelling round the Mediterranean coast, the tourist will be exposed to considerable variation in standard and quality of care available in emergency. It is important to carry the EHIC health card to access reciprocal services where they apply and acquire travel health insurance protection for extra protection for general travel in the region. Distances to good private and state emergency care may be considerable and ambulance transportation limited.

Baltic and Black Sea Cruising

Large and small ship cruising round the Baltic and Black Seas attracts elderly travellers. If illness or trauma befalls passengers, there is recourse to the ship doctor who will off-load seriously ill or injured patients at the next port of call or by helicopter rescue to the nearest land hospital. Most of the shores of the Baltic belong to the EU countries Denmark, Sweden, Germany, Lithuania, Latvia and Estonia which have reciprocal emergency health arrangements with the UK. Travel health insurance cover will be required for repatriation if needed.

Russia. Most Baltic ships call into Leningrad and the traveller will be dependent on the Russian health care system. Russia has a very low standard of compulsory state funded healthcare compared to Western Standards. Healthcare is theoretically free and available to all citizens but patients say doctors, nurses and surgeons routinely demand payments - even bribes - from those they treat. Medical staff are adequately trained; however there is a lack of funding and medical equipment. Old Soviet ways still prevail leading to inequality. Russia has more physicians, hospitals, and health care workers than almost any other country in the world on a per capita basis, but since the collapse of the Soviet Union, the health of the Russian population has declined. Medical care in Russia is among the worst in the industrialized world. A 2000 World Health Organization report ranked Russia's health system 130th out of 191 countries. There are private medical facilities in the cities.

Case History. A 70 year old lady on an inland tour from a cruise ship berthed in Leningrad ate infected ice cream and became ill. Vomiting and with diarrhoea the hotel doctor dispatched her in the middle of the night in a van to an infectious disease unit in the city. It was surrounded by high walls with an electrified fence and entry gates. Admitted to a ward and prostrated by loss of fluid and electrolytes she was stripped, placed under a shower and hosed down with cold water. None of the staff spoke English and she had been admitted without money, passport and day clothes. A doctor prescribed mist. mag. Trisil et pulv. given to the patient on the hand of a nurse and forced into her mouth at regular intervals. Told by signs that her group had continued on their tour, she had a dreadful, neglected few days before making a recovery. The nurses expected bribes for bed-making and provision of bedpans. Only the intervention of the tour group leader eased her discharge.

Consideration

- Adequate travel health insurance is a must for visitors but will only provide the best available care which can be of poor quality.

- "Informal payments" may be expected for basic nursing care.

- Health facilities vary greatly within cities and across the country

Bulgaria, Georgia, Romania, Russia, Turkey, and Ukraine. These countries border the Black Sea with health care provision for tourists akin to that described previously and often of very low standard. The Crimean coast has long been renowned for its health spas and there is a thriving medical tourism industry. Travel health insurance is vital to access private facilities and ensures speedy repatriation. (See comments by country)

Caribbean Islands.

Air/cruise holidays bring many elderly travellers, to Caribbean Islands. About 20 million tourists visit the islands annually most arriving by ship.(16) and a hundred ships cruise round them in the European winter season. They can disgorge 12,000 passengers daily on the quays of large and small islands and overburden medical resources. Although each ship carries a medical and nursing staff, if serious medical or traumatic incident occurs on board, the patient will be disembarked at the next port of call whenever possible. 17Local medical and onward repatriation facilities may be incapable of meeting demand.18Medical care can also be of the variable standard Some islands have modern hospitals with good diagnostic and investigative expertise, but there may be a dearth of nurses, doctors, infrastructure and resources.

Health care provision differs from island to island depending upon size, population, and wealth and is usually provided to visitors on a private basis. There is an increasing tendency for elderly tourists, faced with high premiums and illness exclusions for current medical problems, to travel without travel health insurance cover. They travel uninsured for conditions most likely to befall them and in emergency, face high medical costs if requiring medical attention or hospitalisation. In emergency seriously ill patients may be transferred from islands to the USA for continuing treatment and be faced with exorbitant fee demands.

Disease infection risk for tourists is not high in the islands. However Dengue fever and malaria infections are increasing .**Guadeloupe and Martinique** confirm an increasing number of cases of Hepatitis is a special risk in **Dominican Republic**. HIV/AIDS remains a problem on many islands Malaria had been eradicated (except in Haiti and Dominican Republic), but there has been a resurgence in tourist frequented islands. **Jamaica, Puerto Rico and Cuba** have recently seen cases and deaths, with reports from **Cayman Islands, the British and American Virgin Islands,**

Cruise ship passengers particularly run the risk of norovirus infection and the afflicted old person may become dehydrated, debilitated and require island hospitalisation. Infected tourists from Dominica were quarantined on arrival in Glasgow in 2007. Badly debilitated sufferers will be disembarked en route, or at departure ports in Jamaica, Puerto Rica and Barbados where they may be quarantined and hospitalised with or without their consent.

Cruise ships carry many elderly passengers who suffer heart attacks and strokes on board and have to be hospitalised at next port of call. Cardiac medical emergencies are most likely to result in premature disembarkation. Many tourists also suffer from trauma during a sojourn in the islands. Road systems are often embryonic, poorly maintained and suffer urban congestion. The unfortunate victim may find that ambulance response may be non existent, or delayed and accident and emergency facilities limited and f short in resources. A shortage of water and poor hygiene is evident inland from many of the ports. In island interiors and hinterland people are poor, live frugally in shanties. Local restaurant and café cuisine and ice cream can be infected. Small coastal resort eating places may offer barracuda and amberjack on the menu and there is a risk of cigatuera poisoning from a neurotoxin in fish which feed off reefs.

Elderly tourists sunbathe on beaches and suffer from sun over-exposure, coral abrasions, swimming and sailing accidents. Quad biking, horse riding and off- road 4x4 vehicle pastimes tempt the senior tourist into unwise activities not contemplated in the home scene. Raft, river and rapid- running result in skin abrasions, lacerations and fractures on islands .Older people, who would never consider such activity in UK, abandon inhibition and in holiday spirit expose themselves to physical hurt ,a major cause of tourist morbidity

In **Barbados**- a prime tour destination for Britons- one million tourists were studied. There were 704 emergency admissions with 26 deaths.14% were due to falls, 4.2 % due to road accident and 300 injuries required emergency medical evaluation/management per million tourists /year.

Case Histories:

1. *In the hinterland of Grenada, two vehicles in front of a hired car were involved in head-on road accident. One passenger was knocked unconscious and had a serious head injury. Many miles and hours from the nearest hospital, emergency aid was distant and over bad roads. There was no ambulance facility. A taxi driver had to be bribed to carry him to the emergency unit in the island capital, the only route to urgent medical care.*
2. *A cruise ship reversed passage to carry a passenger with a severe myocardial infarction back to Barbados, which had better medical facilities than the nearer small island and the next destination. After a top speed*

six hour sail, the patient died en route to the hospital after disembarkation. Immediate intensive care hospital attention might have saved him.

Most islands have medical facilities which expect payment at the time of service, and there can be delays in accessing insurers if communications are poor. The islands usually have radiographic facilities but may not have MRI scanners and have limited laboratory services. To access these may mean a journey to another island, or to the mainland of North or South America. Serious cases in Trinidad are often transferred to Venezuela and in the American Virgin Islands, such as the tourist Mecca of **St .Thomas**, to the USA. Uninsured or inadequately insured patients may face unanticipated very expensive hospital and medical costs. The EHIC card is applicable in all French overseas departments (**Martinique, Guadeloupe, and French Guiana**) as they are part of the EEA, but not in Aruba

Very ill patients who are transferred to small islands may face prolonged delay in air transfer to units with better facilities, due to dearth of land and air transport and weather vagaries. Hurricane, landslide, volcanic eruption and tremor make roads impassable on many of these islands, which are mountainous or subject to flooding. The possibility of prolonged evacuation to modern medical and nursing facilities if injured or ill is not considered by British tourists, accustomed to prompt NHS ambulance transfer and emergency response.

Considerations

- Pretravel consultation should bring potential health care shortcomings to the attention of travellers to the Caribbean.

- High technological cardiac care and rehabilitative resources are unlikely to be available in many islands, a consideration for travellers suffering from chronic ill health.

- Island pharmacies have a limited range of pharmacological products. Replacement medications may not be available in the Caribbean.

- Water and food contamination should be kept in mind on small islands and in island hinterlands. Tourists should anticipate infection problems and remember the adage that ingested food should be boiled, cooked, peeled or rejected if they are to avoid food and water borne infection.

- Influenza and Pneumococcal immunisation, Hepatitis A vaccination is recommended and yellow fever vaccination is necessary for those calling in to Venezuelan ports.

- Antimalarial prophylaxis is necessary for those travelling on ships with landfalls in Central and South America.

- Dental treatment is best avoided to decrease risk of hepatitis

- Safety of vehicular transport and availability of seat belts should be considered

- Local evacuation, hospital and emergency resources need consideration

Summary

A visit to Caribbean islands is associated with low health risk, but trauma, or illness can expose the tourist to lower standards of evacuation, immediate and continuing care than that expected in the UK.

Middle East travel

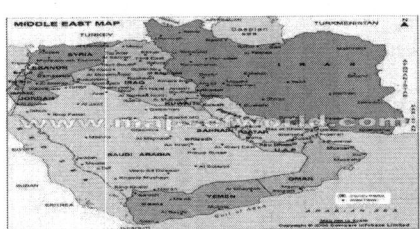

Sun, sand and antiquities attract elderly tourists to the Middle East. Along the eastern littoral of the Mediterranean and the Red Sea there has been a proliferation of holiday resorts. Sanitation and health care resources are not always commensurate with expansion of tourist facilities. In this part of the developing world access to clinics, hospitals and health professionals can be limited and the quality of resource and emergency care variable. From Sharm el Sheik to Damascus, Eilat to Dubai aged tourists embark on the cultural trail through this developing world. New hotels and beach facilities are often dependent upon primitive infrastructure and the services of personnel living in squalor. The risk to western visitors from infection and trauma is high and when overtaken by illness or injury, immediate health care may be unavailable or inadequate.(See previous section on the Mediterranean littoral

Facilities, resources and access can be problematic or absent in this part of the world. Recent terrorist attacks in popular resorts have exposed weaknesses in emergency response and casualty care systems. State run hospitals and clinics are often under-resourced and of variable standard with private establishments scarce and expensive. Sea cruisers and elderly people wandering historic sites are exposed to trauma on poor roads, water sports accidents, injury from terrorist explosions and illness from ingestion of infected water and food. Passengers disembark for tours of the Pyramids and ancient Greek, Roman and Phoenician cities. Day time temperatures spiral to high extremes in the Middle East and archaeological sites become arid ovens by midday, which can desiccate the unwary. Older people are at greater risk of stroke in this situation. They can also become confused when dehydrated and may not react rationally to fluid loss, electrolyte imbalance and fail to recognise the need to rehydrate.

The local population may have primitive sanitation scant water supply and vegetable and fruit produce may have been fertilised by" night soil". Water in hotels and restaurants may be contaminated and the risk of gastro-enteric infection is high. River cruises along the River Nile bring a high risk of enteric infection from contaminated water and elderly people run a greater risk from dehydration in high ambient temperatures. Tourists forget that the on-board water may have been drawn from the river .Most passengers forget or ignore the risk of infection from salads, ice and unbottled water ingested on board and the attrition rate of illness is high. In high ambient temperatures dehydration and electrolyte imbalance can result from the resultant diarrhoea with older people likely to be more severely affected. Treatment will depend on the facilities of a local hospital limited in human and equipment resources.[19]

Case history. *On a bus tour round the sights of Syria only two out of 24 elderly tourists were fit to continue the tour one morning. The others all had severe gastro-intestinal illness. The probable cause of infection was chicken they had eaten at a barbeque lunch organised on a previous day visit to an isolated crusader castle perched on a hill in the desert. No one had considered how the Bedouin had prepared the chicken and vegetables in this waterless unhygienic location. There were no toilets or hand washing facilities. The devoured infected poultry brought dire retribution with none of the infected able to travel onward and two travellers who had become dehydrated required hospital care.*

Case History *An elderly lady visiting the Valley of the Queens in Egypt on a broiling hot cloudless day ,with reflections from the amphitheatre of rocks and sand escalating ambient environmental temperature. Dehydrated, confused and stumbling about, when given a bottle of precious and expensive water she squandered the fluid by pouring the content of the bottle over over-heated feet rather than down her throat.*

Exploration of historic sites usually means traverse of rough, unpaved locations and manoeuvres over rocks, and crudely hewn walkways. A stumble may result in fall and fracture with hospitalisation in the arthritic and older people with poor balance.Emergency aid may be distant, evacuation problematic and health professional help variable and limited. Cruise ships plying their trade in local waters tend to be small with very limited health facilities and doctors from the former soviet empire. They are restricted in passenger health support and off load the ill and injured at the nearest health facility, which may not meet western standards of care. Passengers rarely realise the limitations of small ship cover and the likelihood of immediate disembarkation to a local health facility if medical mishap occurs.

Exposure to the warm waters of the Red Sea and Persian Gulf can bring trauma within and outwith the water and from over-exposure to fierce sun. If injury occurs immediate casualty care response may be rudimentary and evacuation difficult and prolonged. Reusable needles syringes and equipment can pose a threat of hepatitis B and HIV infection and blood supplies may be suspect in some locations. The sporty often also fail to arrange the additional health insurance cover advisable for their physical activities. Older tourists also undertake sub aqua diving and para gliding, riding and other sporty pursuits at these venues forgetting that the small print in their insurance policies will exclude such activity and they will not be covered in the event of accident.

Considerations

- UK health professionals should advise on potential health risks and remind of differences in emergency support likely to be encountered.

- Tourists should ensure adequate health insurance protection and remember that cover only provides the best health care available which may not meet tourist expectations.

- Travellers should be aware of health hazards they might meet,take precautions, particularly against gastrointestinal infection and seek appropriate vaccination.

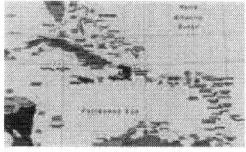

Summary There is a high risk to health in travel through the Middle East from trauma, infection particularly gastro-intestinal disease. High ambient temperatures bring the risk of dehydration and sun burn. Quality of emergency care facilities varies from country to country and within the country. Good medical aid may be distant and evacuation difficult and lengthy.There are good private facilities in the main tourist centres but these are sparse in the hinterlands and rural locations. Private travel health protection is paramount.

Health Care in North and South America

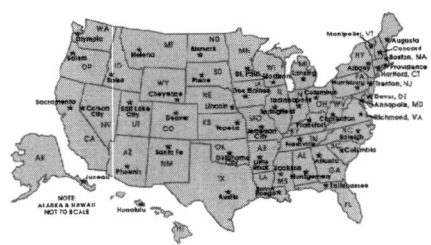

United States of America

Case History. A 68 year old woman had a severe stroke on a cruise ship sailing in the Caribbean, with a home port in Florida. She had suffered a mild stroke 2 years previously and was not covered by her travel health insurance for any recurrence or symptoms of cardio and cerebro-vascular disease. On admission to hospital in the USA she was very ill and required lengthy intensive health care and rehabilitation. The admission contract made with the family made them responsible for all financial costs. Treatment, hospital management and repatriation expenses bankrupted them.

This is not an uncommon case with ill travellers who are hospitalised in America. The need for all visitors to have comprehensive and adequate health insurance is crucial and should be emphasised at pretravel clinic consultations. Tourists should only venture there certain of personal health insurance protection with close scrutiny of small print clauses and exceptions to cover. Failure to secure health cover, or travel with insufficient protection or exclusions for past medical conditions may prove disastrous. Ill tourists to the United States are exposed to very high fees inherent in the private health care sector. 20

The case history illustrates a problem faced by many Americans. The U.S. only holds 37th place in the WHO list of top countries for quality health care services, despite being the highest spender. 45 Million US residents have no health coverage at all. 25 million people who are underinsured spend more than 10% of their income on out of pocket medical costs. Underinsured, they are particularly vulnerable, as are unwary tourists. Until a health catastrophe occurs, visitors are often unaware of exposure to health risk.

Canada. Health care in Canada is delivered through a publicly-funded health care system, which is mostly free at the point of use and has most services provided by private entities. A system of high quality, for residents ,visitors have to make private arrangements in emergency, with costs not dissimilar to the USA and adequate insurance cover is essential. Canada is a very large country with vast distances between towns and villages in the interior. Doctor's surgeries can be a hundred miles apart and distance and weather can delay immediate access to emergency health care for tourists to the hinterland. 21.

High quality emergency medical care is available in North America providing the patient is insured. In the absence of this protection there can be very long waits to access A. & E. units and fees can be extortionate if hospital admission is required. In rural areas distance can delay urgent admission especially if weather conditions prevent emergency flights.

South America draws the adventurous traveller, with unique cultural and scenic attractions enticing the tourist.to Chile, Bolivia and Peru The intrepid traveller needs to journey in robust good health to overcome the rigours of the route. Diverse geography, large distances, tenuous communications, high altitude ,temperature extremes, infection and trauma can affect the tourist who should anticipate health problems22

Case history. In an elderly group of travellers in Chile, a man developed a myocardial infarction and a lady a rasping cough which went on into pneumonia. In pain he waited three hours to see the only doctor and as the sole ambulance was in use, he had to be transported by bus back to Calambra hospital 3 1/2 hours away. After several hours waiting to be seen there and an ECG., which confirmed the infarction, he was advised that facilities were so inadequate in the hospital that he should return to his hotel. He had travelled 7 hours to have the diagnosis confirmed but remained untreated. He was eventually repatriated back to the UK by air. The woman deteriorated despite antibiotic therapy. With poor investigative local resources she was forced to abandon her holiday and return to Santiago. UK tour operators did not provide the ongoing support that they inferred and intercontinental communication between insurance companies, tour operators and patients was desultory and anxiety provoking, adding psychological trauma to the scene.

Medical emergency and evacuation problems are likely to prevail in impoverished, undeveloped and distant tourist locations in rural parts of South America. Even with adequate health insurance cover, protection can only provide what is available. Accessibility and quality of service varies across the regions. State of the art private facilities may be located in the big cities, but an embryonic health service with limited facilities is likely in the rural scene. Land evacuation is protracted and sometimes impracticable. Prompt air evacuation is not assured for cardiac and respiratory conditions as helicopter and small aeroplane transfer is rarely practicable.

A trip across the continent traverses the backbone of the Andes. Such a journey requires preplanning, physical stamina and endurance to accomplish successfully. It is now being undertaken by middle aged and elderly people some of whom are frail and chronically ill. Travel agencies do not adequately inform customers of the physical and psychological ardour of this itinerary. Most are poorly informed about the risk of prolonged travel at altitude, when much of the time spent in Bolivia and Peru will occur at 4,000 metres altitude and higher. Older and chronically ill, at risk, travellers contemplating such a trip should seek a pretravel health consultation.

Chileand Bolivia. Geothermal areas are unguarded. Unwary visitors get scalded from superheated mud pools and fall through silica encrustments into boiling water and steam caverns. First aid attention may be a day of car travel away. Tourists rarely appreciate the health risk of Acute Mountain Sickness (AMS) and fail to recognise headache and vomiting threatens the onset of pulmonary and cerebral oedema and death. Those with chronic cardiac and respiratory problems are over-challenged and may be precipitated into cardiovascular and respiratory failure. Adverse health effects are compounded for those travelling over the border from Chile in to Bolivia, with average travel altitude over3500 metres and passes climbing to 5000 metres and more.

Onward travel in a developing country with poor hygiene facilities exposes the traveller to gastroenteritis and added fluid and electrolyte loss can add to dehydration. Sanitation can be basic, hand washing difficult and food exposed to flies and contamination. The thin air at high altitude poorly screens the suns harmful ultraviolet light rays and solar burn is a constant .Roads are very bad, vehicle related trauma is far more frequent than in the UK. with emergency aid often many hours away.

Recommendations

- Travellers should be aware that if affected by AMS. in these remote areas will face a long, rough trip to lower altitude with evacuation taking up to 24 hours. This delay could prove fatal.

- Prophylaxis with a carbonic anhydrase inhibitor reduces the likelihood of Acute Mountain Sickness.200 mg. of acetazoleamide should be taken 24 hours before exposure to an altitude of 3000 metres and continued daily while at high altitude.

- Be aware that some policies from insurance companies exclude cover if one ventures above 12,000feet.

- Consider that first aid and medical care will be delayed and limited, which may be a decisive factor in survival following infection, medical mishap or trauma.

- Precautions are required against enteric infection.

- Uvl screen filters should be used.

- Tourist transport often carries oxygen in cylinders for people with AMS. It is a wise precaution to ensure there is a cylinder on board before departure.

- Big towns such as Sucre have private medical clinics and La Paz has good access to well equipped private medical units for those who have travel health insurance protection.

Peru. A 2000 World Health Organization report ranked Peru health system 130th out of 191 countries. Lake Titicaca is a magnet for many tourists at over 3,000metres AMS may prevail and its storm-tossed waters can cause motion sickness. Proceeding eastwards and down from the altiplano mosquitos can be a problem. The tourist mecca of Cusco-3,000 metres alt.-is mosquito free, the train however travels down the gorge into the jungle and exposure to malaria transmitting insects. Tourists in shorts with bare arms are often bitten at the ruins in Machu Picchu, in the local town and on the train. They fail to consider prior antimalarial medication or the use of mosquito repellents.

Considerations At pretravel health consultations:-

Health professionals should:-

- deter those with chronic conditions e.g. COAD, the frail elderly, the anaemic, a history of deep vein thrombosis and pulmonary embolism, from setting out on such a trip

Travellers should:-

- Consider pretravel health consultation.

- Seek prophylaxis for malaria and altitude sickness

- Carry, Mosquito repellent protection, anti motion sickness medication, lip salve, first aid kit, water sterilising tablets, large water bottle.

- Anticipate long, arduous land and air journeys

- Assume water, salads, uncooked food to be contaminated unless certain of source.

- If past history includes heart attack, stroke, COAD, immuno-suppression, carefully consider the wisdom of travel.

This is a high health risk part of the world. The older traveller and particularly those with pre-existing illness should consider risk of gastro-intestinal infection, trauma, malaria, acute mountain sickness, solar irradiation and the fatigue of long distance travel in arid , harsh environment. Medical aid may be a day away with no prospect of emergency air evacuation and land transportation is scarce

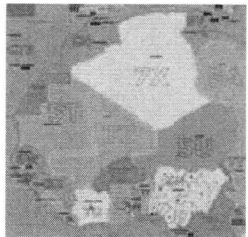

Health Care in West Africa

The west coast of Africa was long known as the Whiteman's Grave because of the high death rate from tropical disease. Countries once shunned by Europeans are now visited in increasing numbers by those intent on accessing winter sunshine. Tourists, apparently protected by comprehensive travel health insurance, often assume that urgent health care needs will be met in medical emergency overseas, as speedily and efficiently as within the NHS. An adverse medical event due to trauma and disease in countries in West Africa however, may expose patients to limited resources and health care and delayed treatment. Insurance companies can only provide the best locally available medical and nursing care. Evacuation and treatment may not equate with that in the developed world. Poor communications, climatic extremes, bad roads and limited transportation threaten delay in emergency hospital access. 23.

Paucity of health professionals, hospitals, and institutional resources determines poor quality of health care provision. Facilities are best in the cities, but up-country and small ports of call often have a rural hinterland, with difficult and distant access to major cities. Traditional medicine, dependent upon herbs and ancient and voodoo practices often ,form part of the primary health care Cruise ships are disgorging passengers into countries fringing the West African coast Standards of emergency care vary considerably from country to country, are often rudimentary and may only be available in the main cities and not in ports.

Common diseases in sub-Saharan countries include cholera, typhoid, pulmonary tuberculosis, anthrax, pertussis, tetanus, chicken pox, yellow fever, measles, infectious hepatitis, trachoma, malaria, and schistosomiasis.

The Gambia - A country with one of the world's lowest per capita income rates, its health care system is rudimentary. There is one teaching hospital in Banjul the capital staffed by consultant specialists mainly from Cuba. There is also an MRC unit in Bakau which specialises in tropical diseases. Both of these are near coastal tourist areas, but are extremely busy, crowded and sleep two patients per bed when under pressure. (24) A few private clinics with limited facilities provide emergency care for the ill or injured tourist, but have scant investigative, or intensive care capacity . The nearest treatment centres are in Dakar, Senegal many hours, drive plus a ferry crossing, away, with transport at a premium and roads often impassable in the wet season. 1 The alternative evacuation route is to Europe, a 6 hours flight, not a viable alternative for a patient with a heart attack, infarction or respiratory emergency as airlines will not fly individuals for a week or ten days after these critical medical incidents. As in all West African countries, malaria is rife.

Senegal, This country is one of the first ports of call for ships leaving the UK in cruises to South Africa and the Far East. If passengers become ill on the Atlantic crossing they may be disembarked here. Private clinics and a few state hospitals are under-resourced, under- doctored and medications may be difficult to acquire. Large disparities still exist in health coverage, with 70% of doctors, and 80% of pharmacists and dentists, living in the nation's capital city, and only 0.1 physicians and 0.4 hospital beds per 1,000 people.

Major health problems include measles and meningitis along with water-related diseases as malaria, trypanosomiasis, onchocerciasis, and schistosomiasis.

Cape Verde Islands. These islands are a port of call for cruise ships on transatlantic crossings. Health facilities are very limited, and some medicines are in short supply, or unavailable. There are hospitals in Praia and Mindelo, with smaller medical facilities elsewhere. Brava and Santo Antão islands no longer have functioning airports so air evacuation in medical emergency is impossible. Malaria occurs in Cape Verde, with risk is mainly limited to the island of Santiago, and highest risk from July to December.

Ghana. Ghana has Government funded health care, with hospitals and clinics also run by religious groups and a few " for-profit" clinics playing a role. Urban centres are well served; however, rural areas often have no modern health care. Patients there rely on traditional African medicine, or travel great distances for care. Ghana experiences the full range of diseases endemic to the region. Private and state facilities are available to tourists in Accra, but are generally poor in the rural scene. As with most West African countries, there is a high health risk from road traffic accident and emergency aid may be delayed, casualty units far distant with limited resources for transfusion and surgery. Travel health insurance companies can negotiate reasonable care for patients in emergency and there are good air connections to Europe.25

Sierra Leone is recovering from a vicious civil war when the infrastructure was damaged. Hospitals and clinics are decayed. Money buys access to what health support is available. Ambulance transferis rare. This is a hazardous place for pedestrians and vehicles and the risk of accidental trauma is high. Emergency admission to a local medical unit is best avoided, but air evacuation depends upon a few direct flights to Europe. Transport is scarce, the roads often dirt tracks and communication between centres fragmented. The few hospitals and clinics are grossly overburdened with the demands of a malnourished destitute population.

The country suffers from epidemic outbreaks of diseases including yellow fever, cholera, Lassa fever and meningitis

Ivory Coast (Cote d'ivoire). In the Ivory Coast there are sharp regional and socioeconomic disparities in health care. There are 12 physicians per 100,000 people. Access to potable water and waste disposal systems is limited in rural areas. The health care system is unable to meet the health care needs of the population, with continuing low ratios of doctors and nurses to patients. Chronic shortages of equipment, medicines, and contribute to overall poor service delivery. In rural areas, health care remains a under the guidance of lineage elders and traditional healers.

Malaria, yellow fever, sleeping sickness, yaws, leprosy, trachoma, and meningitis are endemic..

Cameroon. Health care for tourists is available in big cities in Cameroon. Simple blood samples are usually analysed in the country,but complex ones go to France. Health care activities are either run as government services, or private services managed by various churches. Modern equipment is needed, with many clinics using outdated equipment. In 2004, there were 7 physicians, 36 nurses, per 100,000 people.

Principal diseases are Malaria, HIV Aids, Tuberculosis, sleeping sickness, cholera, dysentery and meningitis. Malaria is prevalent in the coastal region, and the forests. Other serious water-borne diseases are schistosomiasis and sleeping sickness, spread by the tsetse fly. Cameroon lies in the yellow fever endemic zone.

Benin. The population depends upon traditional medical practices- voodoo doctors -when in clinical need. There are a few conventional clinics and hospitals accessible to tourists. There were only 6 physicians and 20 nurses per 100,000 people in 2004. Most serious epidemic diseases have been brought under control Yaws has been almost totally eradicated in the north. Yellow fever has almost disappeared. Cholera cases are now rare.

Sao Tome and Principe. These are small islands lying on the equator off the coast of Africa, an attractive port of call for cruise ships. Medical care is extremely limited. The main health facility is the Ayres Menezes Hospital, located on the island of Sao Tome. Most doctors and hospitals expect payment in cash, regardless of whether the traveller has travel health insurance. Serious medical problems require air evacuation to a country with state-of-the-art medical facilities. Flights are limited and rarely fly direct to Europe. Malaria remains a health risk.

Gabon. In Gabon health facilities remain inadequate, particularly outside the Libreville area. The government provides nearly all health care services. The internationally known Albert Schweitzer hospital is located in Lambaréné. Evacuation and repatriation for the ill or injured tourist is likely to b Malaria, sleeping sickness, tuberculosis, and other infectious diseases are widespread.e delayed and emergency care extremely limited.

Togo. Medical services include treatment centres with services free except at the clinic at the hospital in Lomé, where patients pay a nominal fee. About 61% of the population have access to health care services. In recent years there have been significant decreases in mortality caused by smallpox, yellow fever, and sleeping sickness.

Yaws, malaria, and leprosy continue to be major medical problems

Namibia. Namibia is a country with high levels of inequality in access to health care resources. The main tourist centres have reasonable private health facilities, but tourists safari up country where health units and resources may be unavailable or limited and evacuation can be prolonged (26) Drinking water outside main cities and towns may be contaminated.

Malaria risk exists in the entire northern third of the country from November to June and along the Kunene river and in Kavango and Caprivi regions throughout the year.

Health services in West Africa:-

- are poorly developed and do not meet the needs of all residents

- vary markedly from country to country

- are particularly poor in rural and coastal areas away from cities.

- may not meet the needs of the ill or injured tourist

- Hospitals and clinics are poorly resourced

- Transport to hospital may be unobtainable

- Yellow fever immunisation is mandatory

- Maximal antimalarial precautions are required

- Travel health insurance will not necessarily bring access to optimal emergency care.

- The risk of traffic related trauma is very high

- Air and land evacuation may not be possible in emergency.

Health Care on Safari

South Africa. At the southern end of west African coast line is Capetown, port of call for many cruise ships and ill passengers are off loaded here. The health system consists of a large public sector and smaller private sector. Health care varies from the most basic primary health care, offered free by the state, to highly specialised hi-tech health services available in the private sector. The public sector is under-resourced and over-used. The enlarging private sector, caters for foreigner visitors and medical tourists seeking top-quality surgical procedures at relatively affordable prices. The private sector also attracts most of the country's health professionals. Medical tourists looking for top-quality surgical procedures at relatively affordable prices are visiting in increasing numbers.

Kenya. Access to health care varies widely throughout the country, determined between rural and urban communities, moneyed elite and the poor. Most facilities are located in Central Province, and few in the border provinces of Western Valley and Nyanza. Prevalence of communicable disease in Kenya is a major factor with HIV, malaria and tuberculosis rife. [27] A large percentage of the population does not seek care despite being ill. 90% of the population in sub-Saharan Africa use traditional medicine as their source of primary healthcare. [28]

Stark disparities are apparent in levels of care, and facility to facility in different regions. Top of the service spectrum are Teaching Hospitals such as Kenyatta National Hospital (KNH)in Nairobi. The next best level of care is found in provincial hospitals, with uneven distribution of health workers between urban and rural areas. Contrast in levels of care is seen in KNH, which offers public and private wards, attended by the same doctors. A patient in the public ward, can expect to spend long hours waiting to be seen, and may be expected to share a bed with another patient. Patients are grouped in large, open, chaotic rooms and afforded no privacy which compares badly with the private ward of the hospital. While both public and private patients receive a reasonable level of care at KNH, the disparity between services offered there and elsewhere can be substantial. The provincial general hospital in Nyeri, for instance demonstrates a major drop in quality of care and resources such as morphine, a basic analgesic [29] can be in short supply.

Zimbabwe. Zimbabwe's health-care system is collapsing. Hospitals face dire shortages of doctors and medical supplies and are unable to undertake basic operations because of shortages of anaesthetics, sutures, and essential supplies. The country is battling one of the world's highest rates of infection of HIV/AIDS, estimated to be killing more than 3000 people weekly. Elective surgery has been abandoned in the central hospitals and even emergency surgery is often dependent on the ability of patients' relatives to purchase drugs, suture materials, and supplies of blood from private sellers. Ambulances are grounded for want of fuel and spare parts. [29] Harare, now has regular outbreaks of cholera.

Consideration.

- Elderly people should be advised to avoid travel in the country until the health care system reaches minimal standards of provision.

- The health care and transportation systems have disintegrated and emergency aid is problematic.

- Travel health insurance cover cannot provide protection in the absence of resources.

Zambia. Services to Zambian nationals are free at rural health centres and urban hospitals .The public health care sector suffers from a severe shortage of doctors, medicine, medical equipment and supplies. Zambia has one of the highest rates of HIV infection, even in hard-hit sub-Saharan Africa. There are limited private facilities for tourists.

Malaria and tuberculosis are major health problems and hookworm and schistosomiasis afflict a large proportion of the population

Namibia. This is a popular safari destination .The country is arid, distances between health centres can be considerable and health care variable. (See previous note on Namibia)

Tanzania. Medical treatment is free or highly subsidized in company clinics and hospitals. Tanzania's national health care system stresses primary care at an affordable cost, but faces an acute shortage of health care workers. Low pay, poor working conditions and limited training programs contribute, worsened by the burden of treating HIV/AIDS and malaria patients, Health standards in Tanzania have declined and care is poor. The public system serves the vast majority of the population, but is chronically underfunded and understaffed. The wealthiest 20% of the population uses the private system, the route followed by the insured ill tourist. 30.31

South Africa. Medical facilities are good in urban areas but can be limited elsewhere. Tourists on safari may find themselves distant from medical aid. Private facilities are good where they exist. Kruger National Park, Mpumalanga and northern KwaZulu-Natal are low risk malaria areas during December-April. Swimming and paddling in stagnant or slow-moving water as there is a risk of contracting bilharzia. (See comment on West Africa)

Considerations.

- Safari travel means long hours in four wheel drive vehicles in a dusty, dry wild environment, in areas where malarial mosquitos thrive.

- Safari visits depend upon early morning and late afternoon trips at a time when mosquitos are active.

- Dry and non air-conditioned camping environs make for dehydration and water sources may be infected.

There is a high risk from infection and trauma and emergency medical aid may be distant of variable quality and ambulance evacuation n on-existent.

Central and east African countries which offer wild animal safaris are high risk destinations for elderly travellers. Infection, trauma, dehydration are likely to befall the older person who may find that emergency medical care is distant and not of optimal quality. Ideally safaris should only be embarked upon by those in robust health. Pretravel health consultation is advised for those with pre-existing health conditions, and vaccine prophylaxis and antimalarial precautions should be taken.

Asia Far East and Antipodes

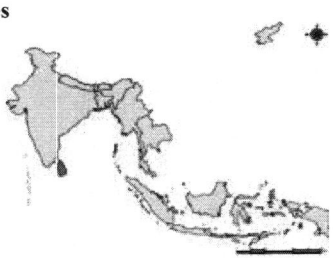

China.

China is undertaking reform of its health-care system to make it more affordable for the rural poor. Chinese medical schools provide training in Western medicine and also instruct in traditional medicine, but relatively few physicians are competent in both areas. In urban hospitals, there may be separate departments for traditional and Western treatment. In county hospitals, however, traditional medicine receives greater emphasis. It depends on herbal treatments, acupuncture, acupressure, moxibustion (the burning of herbs over acupuncture points) and "cupping" of skin, with heated bamboo believed to be most effective in treating minor and chronic diseases. Traditional treatments may be used for more serious conditions as well, particularly for such acute abdominal conditions as appendicitis, pancreatitis, and gallstones, a consideration for foreign visitors who become ill far from major hospital centres.

Western style medical facilities with international staff are available in Beijing, Shanghai, Guangzhou and a few other large cities. Hong Kong has excellent private facilities. Many other hospitals in major Chinese cities have so-called V.I.P. wards or gaogan bingfang. with reasonably up-to-date medical technology and skilled physicians. They provide medical services to foreigners and have English-speaking doctors and nurses.

India A universal health care system is run by the constituent states. Government hospitals, some of which are among the best hospitals in India, provide treatment at taxpayer expense hospitals, either free or at minimal charges. There is a large private sector in cities and tourist areas .Emergency transportation to hospital can prove a daunting procedure in much of rural, India, a consideration elderly tourists should keep in mind. (See chapter on medical tourism)

Japan. The Government provides healthcare services, with the patient accepting responsibility for 30 % of the bill. Japan has excellent hospitals and clinics, and provides highly-technical, state of the art equipment. Patients are free to select physicians or facilities of their choice. Due to large numbers of people visiting hospitals emergency access is an issue in some units and a particular problem in Tokyo. In 2007 14,000 emergency patients were rejected at least three times by Japanese hospitals before getting treatment .Some healthcare in Japan is provided free for expatriates and foreigners. The Japanese have no 'family-doctor' system and medical ethics and bedside manners are not strong points with health professionals.

Malaysia The country offers a comprehensive network of hospitals and clinics, with 88.5 percent of the population living within three miles of a public health clinic or private practitioner. (See chapter 12 on medical tourism)

Nepal. The health-care delivery network in Nepal is poorly developed. Government-operated health-care delivery system consists of hospitals and health centres with very basic facilities. Health-care practices in rural areas often depends upon the medicine man or shaman as well as Ayurvedic treatment Allopathic (modern) medicine and quality of care is poor. There are private medical facilities in Kathmandhu. Diarrhoeal disease is a major public health problem. There is high risk of road accident trauma.Evacuation may be difficult and protracted with limited air transport and tenuous road movement. In the higher valleys, patients may have to be carried to hospital on a Sherpa's back.32-33

Infection risk is considerable with high endemicity of malaria, food and water borne disease such as diarrhoea,Typhoid, paratyphoid fever, giardiasis, amoebiasis, helminthiosis),kala-zarrRabies,hepatitis B.There is also a risk from the effects of high altitude inducing acute mountain sickness.

Considerations

- Malaria prophylaxis

- Prophylaxis with acetazolamide for high altitude exposure

- Assumption that all water is contaminated and use of water sterilising tablets.

- Consideration of limited emergency care and protracted evacuation and hospital access

South East Asia

IndonesiaThe level of health care in Bali varies from local clinics and hospitals, to foreign run clinics such as SOS International. Small urban clinics can handle simple injuries. Each district in Bali has a hospital located in the main town, however Sanglah in Denpasar is the only one capable of dealing with really major operations and patients are transferred here from elsewhere on the island.

Thailand . The health care system relies heavily on specialized medicine. The Thai Government has developed a universal health care programme whereby everybody gets treatment at public hospitals for a standard fee per visit. If foreigners have a medical problem while in Thailand, a few hospitals of good reputation, cater for foreign patients.with Bumrungrad Hospital being popular. Bangkok General Hospital and its affiliates Samitivej Hospital and Bangkok Nursing Home Hospital, are also commended. Certain hospitals have been actively seeking medical tourists to visit Thailand and now up to 60% of patients at Bumrungrad Hospital and 40 % at Samitivej Hospital are foreigners. (See chapter on medical tourism)

Summary

Large variations in health care occur across the region with some countries having excellent resources and catering for medical tourism. Congested roads and poor transportation result in high road traffic accident risk and trauma in many countries. Emergency transportation can be limited. Travel health insurance cover essential. There is a high likelihood of gastrointestinal infection and malaria in many of these countries.

Antipodes

Australia. Australia has a highly commended medical care system. The Australian Government has signed Reciprocal Health Care Agreements (RHCA) with the government of the United Kingdom which entitles British visitors to limited subsidised health services for medically necessary treatment while visiting Australia.*This covers* any ill-health or injury which occurs while in Australia and requires amedical attention. The The Royal Flying Dotor Service provides and excellent service to rural many rural areas .34 but emergency aid can be delayed due to adverse weather.35A resident of UK is entitled to the following for any ill-health or injury requiring treatment:-

- free treatment as a public in-patient or outpatient in a public hospital
- subsidised medicines under the Pharmaceutical Benefits Scheme

- Medicare benefits for out-of-hospital medical treatment provided by doctors through private surgeries and community health centres.

Medical treatment can be accessed through private doctors' surgeries and community health centres. Doctors at these practices charge for their services by charging Medicare direct or presenting a bill for payment by the patient which is then reimbursed by Medicare.If treated as a public patient in a public hospital, treatment is free on display of passport or reciprocal health care card to staff at the hospital.Medicare will not cover:

- medicines not subsidised under the Pharmaceutical Benefits Scheme
- dental work and allied health services
- accommodation and medical treatment in a private hospital
- accommodation and medical treatment as a private patient in a public ambulance services
- home nursing
- physiotherapy, occupational therapy, therapy, eye therapy, chiropractic services, podiatry glasses and contact lenses, hearing aids

New Zealand. The New Zealand health system functions on the Anglo-American model of care, with emergency care in the prehospital setting being conducted by paramedics.There are reciprocal arrangements with the|UK.and WHO rates the system highly.

The World Health Organization in 2001 ranked the health systems of 191 nations. France and Italy took top spots and Australia, New Zealand, Canada and the UK rating highly with Germany on most measures of performance, including quality of care and access to it.

Extreme latitudes Arctic and Antarctic

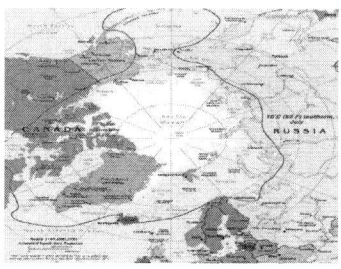

80,000 tourists per year visit the Falklands and Antarctica and a significant number visit the Arctic on cruise ships varying in size from small, ice-strengthened vessels, to massive cruise liners which combine several days cruising around the Falklands with South Georgia and Antarctica. Greenland , the Svalbard peninsula and Spitzbergen. Larger cruise ships have the health facilities of modern luxury ships.Small ones may not have an on board doctor and irrespective of size they will off load ill or injured passengers in the Falkland Islands if cruising southern seas and to Svalbard and the main land in the Arctic.Helicopter rescue is limited by range in the Arctic and patients have to be air evacuated from Svalbard to Tromso and from Greenland to Denmark for intensive care. Denmark and Norway, the nearest mainland countries to Greenland and Svalbard. They have very good health facilities with UK reciprocation. 27

Some land-based tourists visit the **Falklands Islands** alone. There are no indigenous diseases or poisonous creatures in the area however, travel to the Falklands usually means coming via South America and travellers are advised to check requirements for each country carefully. The water supply is safe and There is a reciprocal health agreement between the UK and Falkland Island Governments which allows free medical treatment for UK residents in the Falklands. This does not cover dental care The reciprocal agreement does not cover medical care in Ascension Island nor in St Helena possible landings en route Medical services are based in the modern, 27 bed, well-equipped King Edward VII Memorial Hospital (KEMH) in Stanley. There are 4 General Practitioners with extended skills, two consultants and 28 nurses, There is 1 radiographer with a range of modern digital plain X-ray equipment,excluding CT and MRI scanner. The pharmacy is well stocked with UK pharmaceuticals .Tourists are strongly advised to bring enough of their regular medication to cover the whole duration of their holiday.36

Given the small size of the hospital, the limited range of diagnostic facilities available and the limited ability to manage intensive care patients, coupled with the lack of complex treatments such as kidney dialysis, it is normal to stabilise a critically ill person and then transfer then to a larger hospital. KEMH has an agreement with the Clinica Aleman in Santiago and and every tourist must be insured to cover this potential cost. "Aerocardal" transport charges in the region of US$ 30,000. Fees of the Clinica Alemana are comparable to a private hospital anywhere in Europe so he cost there could be in the region of $40,000 US or more. The RAF normally will not consider transferring a tourist as a patient even if they are UK passport holders. During the tourist season, October- March, doctors are accustomed to dealing with overseas hospitals, transfers and insurance companies. Ships leave from Stanley to cruise the Antarctic peninsula and islands a four day sail away from the nearest aid in the Falklands. Evacuation is nor practicable and emergency care will depend on the resources of the ship. There are small village clinics in Greenland villages and Svalbard has a small hospital unit. Serious conditions have to be evacuated by small fixed wing aircraft, an expensive undertaking. Local Governments are now insisting that visitors have repatriation insurance in place before arrival

Consideration The standard of medical care in the Falklands is broadly similar to the UK but tourists must bear in mind the limitations imposed by the size of the hospital, range of specialists and the limited range of diagnostic equipment available.

Case History

On a sea crossing from the North Cape of Norway to Greenland an elderly woman was wheel chair dependent and required help from her husband with all basic needs. The husband had a severe heart attack and had to be airlifted by helicopter, operating at its maximal range, to the nearest hospital in Norway. Bereft of assistance in daily living the care of the wife became a major problem for crew who were not allowed to touch passengers far less offer intimate care and a harassed medical/nursing staff struggling to support with passengers with norovirus infection. She had to be airlifted to the mainland by small aeroplane in an exercise which had to be funded by the patient as she was uninsured.

Elderly potential travellers to Antarctica and the Arctic should organise a pretravel health consultation. Travel health insurance protection is essential with adequate cover for repatriation. They should be aware that emergency aid may be many hours and in bad weather days away.

References

1 McIntosh I 1991 Travel Induced Illness Scot. Med. 11.4 14-15
2 www.nhs.uk/NHSEngland/.../EHIC/Pages/Introduction.aspx
3 Honor M. Medical care for visitors to France. 2008Brit.Trav.Health Assoc J.10.20-21
4 Mackay I Primary Care services with the EU. 2007. Brit.Trav.Health AAssoc. IX,10-15

5 Mackay I Health care on a European river cruise.2010 Brit.Trav.Health Assoc.J 15.26-9

6 Rhisel R. Pay as you go in Romania 2010 Brit.Trav.Health Assoc.J 16.60

7. Gaál, P., Rekassy, B., and Healy, J. Health Care Systems in Transition: Hungary. Copenhagen: European Observatory on Healthcare Systems, 1999.

8 Orosz, E. and Hollo, I. 'Hospitals in Hungary: The story of stalled reforms,' Eurohealth, vol. 7, num. 3, Autumn 2001.

9 Gaál, P. Study of the Hungarian Health Care System. Civitas, 2002.

Bulgaria Orosz, E., and Burns, A. The Healthcare System in Hungary. Paris: Organisation for Economic Co-operation and Development, 2000.

10 Shannon C. Irvine F and B Analysis of Hungary' Health Care System www.civitas.org.uk/nhs/download/Hungary.

11 Popova S Feschieva, N The state of primary medical care in Bulgaria Journal of Public Health 1995 17, 1. 6-10

12 McCarthy M Serbia rebuilds and reforms its health care system The Lancet, 2007 Volume 369, I0,

13 Croatia European Observatory on Health Care SystemsAMS 5001891 (CRO)CARE 04 01 02

14 Melrose A Health Care Round the Mediterranean2009 Brit.Trav.Health Assoc.J21-23

15 McIntosh I Health care and security for travellers to Middle east.2005 Brit.Trav.Health Assoc.J26-27

16 Mackay I Health Care Caribbean style Brit.Trav.Health AssocJ. 11.9-10

17 McIntosh I Cruise ship facilities 2007 Brit.Trav.Health Assoc.J10.10-12

18 McIntosh I health and safety on cruise ships2007 Brit.Trav.Health Assoc.J 10-15

19 McIntosh I Health care and security for travellers to the Middle east2005 Brit.Trav.Health Assoc.J

20 Mackay I Health Care in the USA. 2009 Brit.Trav.Health Assoc.J13.16-17

21 Bailley R. Rural health service in north Saskatchewan2007. X 23

22 MackayII Travel and Health across South America.2007 Journal of BTHA, X, 19-21

23 Melrose A. Health care for visitors and residents in west Africa.2011 Brit.Trav Health Assoc J 16 25-27

24 Dalton K Health care in the Gambia Brit.Trav Health Assoc J 2010 16.23

25 Eyob Zere, Custodia MandlhateEquity in health care in Namibia: developing a needs-based resource allocation formula using principal components analysis Int J Equity Health. 2007; 6: 3

26 2whohgana@gha.fro.who.intUNICEF, 2008

27 Wamai, RG. (2009). "The health system in Kenya: Analysis of the situation and enduring challenges." JMAJ. 52(2): 136.

28.Kareru, PG, Kenji, GM, Gachanja, AN, Et al. (2007). "Traditional medicines among the Embu and Mbeere peoples of Kenya." Afr. J. Trad. CAM. 4(1): 75.

30.Mwww.worldlifeexpectancy.com/country-health-e. Tanzania health system e.

31 http://www.nationsencyclopedia.com/Africa/Tanzania-HEALTH.html#ixzz1EJuipEOU

32 Mackay I Nepal, the tourist view of the health scene. 2004 J.Brit. Health Assoc 5 ,35-6

33 Kharal PM Travel Medicine in Nepal 2004J Brit. Trav Health Assoc. 5.33-4

34 McIntosh I Royal flying doctor service of Austraklia. 2006 Brit. Trav.heralth Assoc J. 7.26-7

35 Mackay I the good Samaritan.response 2008 Brit. Trav Health Assoc.J. 8.14-16

36 Diggle R.Falkands health care.Journal of Brit.Trav.Health Assoc.J XI, 2008

Iain B. McIntosh

Chapter 14
The Adventurous Older traveller

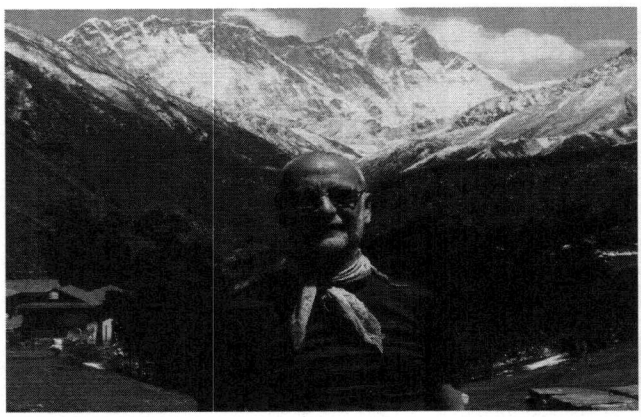

The population of the UK is ageing.[1]Over the last 25 years the percentage of the population aged 65 and over increased from 15 per cent in 1984 to 16 per cent in 2009, an increase of 1.7 million people. By 2034, 23 per cent of the population is projected to be aged 65 and over. The fastest population increase has been in the number of those aged 85 and over, the "oldest old". In 1984, there were around 660,000 people in the UK aged 85 and over. Since then the numbers have more than doubled reaching 1.4 million in 2009. By 2034 the number of people aged 85 and over is projected to be 2.5 times larger than in 2009, reaching 3.5 million and accounting for 5 per cent of the total population.[1]

Figure 1

Population trends in the UK by age group (source: Office of National Statistics)

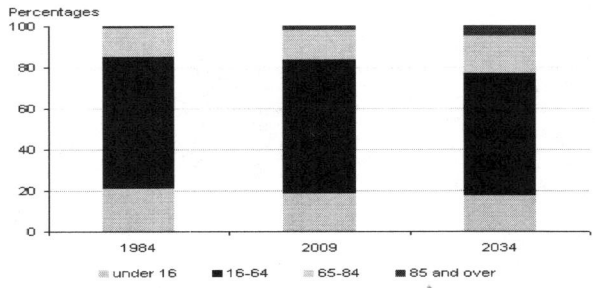

The most numerous five year age groups at the 2001 census were the 5-year group born in the years 1946–51 (the post–World War II baby boom); the baby boom born a generation later in 1966–71 (the largest group of all); and a more modest boom a generation after that, born in 1986–91. The 1946–51 group reaches retirement age from 2006 onwards (women from 2006 and men from 2011), and the sudden increase in the number of people claiming the state pension has led politicians and political commentators to fear a "pensions crisis". UK figures released by the ONS (Office for National Statistics)2 report that by the end of 2011, pensioners will outnumber children for the first time. In 2010, 11.3 million drew a state pension. By 2031 there will be 15 million pensioners even though the pension age will have increased to 66 for men and women after 2024.

Although health expectancy has not improved at the same rate as life expectancy3 older people can currently look forward to better health in old age than did those in previous generations. Although there are currently fears about future pension provision, many of today's retired people are in a better financial state than their forebears. Attitudes to ageing and what might be deemed appropriate behaviour for older people have also changed a great deal, so that many who would have been reaching for their pipes and slippers or doing nothing more active than a little gentle gardening in previous generations are now travelling abroad to ever more exotic destinations and taking part in sport and other extreme physical activities. The author has continued to enjoy such pursuits as mountain trekking and white water rafting since reaching the age of 60, Sir Ranulph Fiennes reached the summit of Everest at the age of 65, and Miin Bahadur Sherchan, a Nepali aged 76 is currently the oldest person to have climbed Everest. Such activities are not however devoid of risk and recently a Nepali aged over 80 died whilst attempting the ascent of Everest.

Physical activity in older people does confer benefits. It has been shown, for example, that physical activity can help a person to cope with mental challenges in the transition period between occupation and retirement4, that weight-bearing exercise in young age and the training continuation in later life may be an important contributor to bone mineral density in middle aged and older people5 and that higher levels of fitness were associated with a lower risk of developing diabetes6. All this, and much more evidence, points to the benefits of pursuing an active lifestyle as age increases. People with higher fitness and higher aerobic capacity have longer life expectancies compared to inactive people. Even at very old ages, regular physical activity results in a lot of benefits, in high quality of life, in independence and longevity.7.

A 67-year old trekker in Nepal

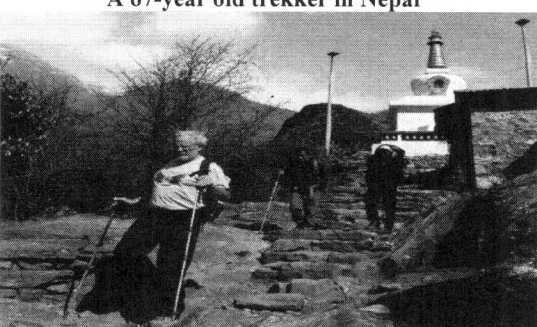

The Older person at high altitude

Some trekking companies place age limits on their clients[8], though the reasons for this are not stated. A study of trekkers in the Solu Khumbu region of Nepal showed no association between age or gender and the incidence of acute mountain sickness (AMS)[9], and this accords with the general experience that age is not a determining factor in the causation of AMS. Indeed, younger trekkers with a higher degree of physical fitness appear to be more at risk of AMS[10]. This may be because they are less inclined to ascend slowly and steadily than are their older counterparts. The presence of pre-existing heart or lung disease does not appear to increase the risk of AMS[10], nor does the decreased sensitivity of the hypoxic ventilatory response found in older people[11].

Acute mountain sickness

Symptoms of AMS

The main symptoms and signs of AMS which AMS have often been compared with having a "hangover" from drinking alcohol, are some or all of the following

* Headache

* Nausea

* Vomiting

* Fatigue

* Loss of appetite

* Dizziness

* Sleep disturbance

Peripheral oedema It is possible for the body to acclimatise to the lower atmospheric pressure, at least up to very high altitude, up to 5800 metres. Higher altitudes than this are unlikely to be encountered by anyone except high altitude climbers.

On initial ascent to high altitude there is an increase in pulmonary ventilation leading to hypocapnia and respiratory alkalosis, compensated for by increased renal excretion of bicarbonate and a bicarbonate diuresis. A rise in heart rate also occurs but the heart rate gradually reduces again as acclimatisation occurs, though at extreme altitude the resting heart rate remains high. Over a longer period erythropoietin secretion increases, leading to increased red blood cell production and a consequent raised haemoglobin concentration and haematocrit. This in turn leads to increased blood viscosity and an increased tendency towards thrombosis.

Acclimatisation can be assisted in the following ways:

* *Gradual slow ascent.* It is often recommended that the net height gain in a day (that is the gain in height from one sleeping place to the next sleeping place ignoring any ups and downs en route) should be no more than 300 metres (1000 feet) per day. This is empirically a safe rate of ascent for almost everyone, though it may be possible for some people to ascend more than this in a day, up to 500 metres a day, without any problems. A few individuals may encounter problems even at a rate of ascent of 300 metres a day. The problem here is that everyone has his or her individual rate of ascent before the body encounters difficulty, and what is the right rate of ascent for most members of a group may produce symptoms in a minority of a group of equally fit and healthy people. On an organised trek, for example, a rate of ascent is usually chosen that is likely to be safe for the group, but even then a few people in a group may develop altitude symptoms. When flying into a high altitude airport symptoms may also occur because in these circumstances there is no time for acclimatisation to occur, though acclimatisation will begin within a few days after arrival

* **Avoiding over-exertion.** Over-exertion is known to increase the chance of developing altitude problems. As has already been stated, youth and fitness do not help to prevent altitude problems. and it has been suggested that older people are less prone to altitude sickness, as they are less likely to over-exert themselves. A useful philosophy on a mountain trek or when walking up to the base camp for a high altitude expedition is that there are no prizes for getting there first. Those who try to set a fast pace to prove their fitness are inviting trouble. A slow and steady pace is what is needed.

* **Adequate fluid intake.** Dehydration has long been thought to increase the chance of developing altitude problems, though the evidence for this no longer appears to be very strong. Fluid loss increases at higher altitudes, partly because of sweating due to exertion and partly due to evaporation from the mouth, throat and lungs due to the drier air and it is important to avoid dehydration by drinking plenty of water whether or not it helps to prevent altitude problems. Tea, coffee and alcohol are diuretics and make the body lose more water than it gains from them. Fluid intake must not be taken to extremes as drinking too much water may cause hyponatraemia.

* **Acetazolamide (Diamox).** The use of acetazolamide, (Diamox) has been shown in many research studies to improve the body's uptake of oxygen by adjusting the body chemistry and to help either to prevent or to treat altitude symptoms. It treats the cause of the problem and does not simply mask its symptoms. Acetazolamide is a carbonic anhydrase inhibitor which causes the kidney to increase its excretion of bicarbonate ions. This causes a metabolic acidosis and in order to compensate for this pulmonary ventilation is increased, increasing excretion of carbonic acid (H_2CO_3, i.e. $H_2O + CO_2$) via the lungs, The result of increased ventilation is that oxygen uptake in the lungs is increased, thereby reducing hypoxia. This cannot be achieved by voluntary hyperventilating without using acetazolamide as this would cause acute respiratory alkalosis with dizziness, paraesthesiae and eventually loss of consciousness. For prevention, acetazolamide should be taken in a dose of 125 to 250 mg twice a day, starting 1 to 2 days before reaching 3000 metres. A higher dose is used for treatment of established symptoms.

A general opinion amongst most altitude experts is that it is not necessary for everyone going to high altitude to take acetazolamide. It is probably best reserved for

* those who have been to altitude previously and did not acclimatise well in spitre of adequate precautions

* treks or expeditions in which the lie of the land means that height gains may exceed the recommended levels per day

* flying in to altitudes of 3000 metres or more with no opportunity to acclimatise

Acetazolamide is a prescription-only drug, therefore it requires a prescription signed by a registered medical practitioner. In addition it does not have a product licence for use for high altitude problems, so that it has to be prescribed "off-licence". Drugs prescribed on a "just in case" basis for travel are not covered by the NHS and the doctor should issue a private prescription. Some GPs are not willing to prescribe acetazolamide for travellers, and if an individual encounters difficulty with this it may be possible to consult a specialist travel clinic. It is also to buy acetazolamide over the counter in some other countries but care must be taken as drugs obtained in this way may be time-expired or counterfeit. Acetazolamide often causes tingling in the hands and feet or elsewhere at the extremities. This is a nuisance if it occurs but is not dangerous. It is also a mild diuretic, and care should be taken to ensure an adequate fluid intake. It is also often said that carbonated drinks taste flat when taking acetazolamide. This who have a drug sensitivity to sulfa drugs should not take acetazolamide, though these drugs are not commonly used nowadays.

Other "altitude remedies" on sale tend to contain little more than aspirin or paracetamol, perhaps with a little caffeine or other ingredients. They may help with headache but they will not help to prevent or treat the real problem.

Prevention of AMS

As the development of AMS signifies that the individual has failed to acclimatise properly the measures likely to assist in its prevention are those listed above as assisting acclimatisation, namely:

* Gradual slow ascent

* Avoiding over-exertion

* Adequate fluid intake

* Acetazolamide 125-250mg twice a day

Treatment of AMS

* It is essential for the affected individual to tell the tour or expedition leader or doctor or some other responsible person that he or she is having problems
* Rest at the same altitude, avoiding any unnecessary exertion and do not ascend higher until symptoms have improved
* Go down to a lower altitude, preferably at least 300 metres, if symptoms do not improve or if they becomebecome worse.
* Acetazolamide 250 mg 2 or 3 times a day

Although age may not predispose to an increased risk of AMS, mountain activities do involve increased levels of exertion which may exacerbate pre-existing cardiac or respiratory problems or render pre-existing but asymptomatic ischaemic heart disease symptomatic. Many older people have musculoskeletal problems such as osteoarthritis of the knees or hips, or foot problems such as bunions, which may not cause serious mobility problems during normal everyday activities but which may be exacerbated by increased levels of exertion involved in trekking. Foot care is especially important for diabetics. Comfortable and previously worn, not brand new, trekking shoes or boots should be worn, with a good tread on the soles to avoid slips and falls. Trekking poles help to reduce the stress on lower limb joints. Two adjustable poles should be used, with the left pole advanced as the right foot advances and vice versa. They should be adjusted in length so that on level ground the elbow is flexed to 900 when the hand grip is held with the poles vertical. They may be shortened for steep uphill slopes and lengthened for steep downhill slopes. Rucksacks should have a waist strap, padded for comfort, with the shoulder straps adjusted so that the weight is distributed between them and the waist strap, and an additional strap linking the two shoulder straps adjusted to reduce tension and dragging on the shoulders.

Climatic and weather conditions in mountain areas can be very variable. It is possible to encounter strong sun, extreme cold, high winds, rain, hail and snow all within the same day. Layered clothing, that can be removed or added to according to the conditions, is essential. The inner layer should be of a material that wicks sweat away from the skin and the outermost layer should be of a breathable, waterproof and windproof material. A good four season sleeping bag is essential, as nights can be very cold, whether camping or staying in lodges. At high altitude there is increased exposure to ultraviolet light (UVL) from the sun, even when there is cloud cover. The presence of snow or pale coloured rock increases this exposure by reflection, and the application of an effective sunscreen to the skin is important, and effective UVL-absorbing sunglasses should be worn to avoid damage to the eyes, preferably with side panels in the presence of snow.

Daytime heat, exertion and low partial pressure of water vapour in the atmosphere at high altitude may result in dehydration, a complication to which older people are more prone[12] and which may also predispose to the development of AMS. It is important to maintain a higher fluid intake in such conditions. It is also important to ensure that only purified or bottled water is used, as the use of local water supplies without purification may lead to diarrhoea, rendering further dehydration likely. In the presence of reduced renal function in older people, dehydration could potentially lead to renal failure. A good guide to an individual's state of hydration is the passage of pale coloured urine.

In the UK's mountain regions such as Scotland, The Lake District and North Wales there is a volunteer mountain rescue service free of charge to those rescued, with free helicopter evacuation when necessary provided by the Royal Air Force, but in other countries there is no such free service. For trekkers in Nepal the cost of a helicopter evacuation can be as much as $2500 per hour[13], and the cost is likely to be similar in most other trekking areas such as South America. The only alternative in Nepal is to be evacuated on the back of a porter, a mule or a yak, which is not only very much slower but involves considerable discomfort for the passenger and possible exacerbation of the medical condition or injury necessitating evacuation. It is therefore essential for the older trekker to ensure that travel insurance covers not only the usual provisions required for travel, including cover for pre-existing medical conditions, but that it also covers the cost of evacuation by helicopter. Travel insurance offered by tour operators is extremely unlikely to offer such cover, and the premium is likely to be high.

Pre-travel advice

* Ensure that the traveller has a reasonable level of physical fitness, e.g. the ability to walk for several hours per day carrying a rucksack

* Ensure that clothing, footwear and other equipment are comfortable and suitable for the activity involved. Tour operators will often provide a suggested kit list

* Advise the traveller about a suitable rate of ascent to avoid developing AMS

* Check that pre-existing medical conditions are stable and controlled and that all necessary medication is carried, with additional spares in case of loss or damage. Check also for other potential problems previously undiagnosed or unreported

* Ensure that the traveller carries an emergency medical kit to cover exacerbations of pre-existing medical conditions and to cater for conditions likely to arise during the trip, such as foot and musculoskeletal problems, diarrhoea and minor injuries

* Ensure that adequate travel and medical insurance has been taken out

The older person in cold climates

Older people have a reduced capacity to regulate body temperature when exposed to cold conditions[14,15]. Cold conditions are encountered at extremes of northern and southern latitudes, for example on Arctic or Antarctic cruises, on winter sports holidays, at high altitude and during the night in desert regions. . In these situations older people may be at risk of hypothermia. Impairment of peripheral circulation may also expose them to the risk of peripheral cold injury. Antarctic cruises tend to attract a high proportion of older people; in one study[16] the mean age of 1057 passengers was 54 years ± 16.5 years, and anecdotal evidence suggests that many passengers on some cruises are well beyond the upper limit of this age range.

Inadequate food intake and wet or inadequate clothing and sleeping bags predispose to cold-related illness. Those who are ill or injured are also more prone to both hypothermia and cold injury, and a variety of medications and the ingestion of alcohol may potentiate the effects of cold. It is important when travelling in conditions in which the air temperature may fluctuate suddenly from warm to cold that travellers are reminded to carry layers of additional insulating clothing, hats and gloves and to put them on as soon as the temperature begins to fall.

Hypothermia

Hypothermia is said to occur when the body core temperature falls below 35°C17. Some mental processes, such as decision making, may already be impaired at this temperature, and excessive shivering may occur. Below this temperature, behaviour becomes inappropriate, clumsiness and confusion occur and, as the body temperature falls lower, there is impairment or loss of consciousness and the shivering stops. When the temperature has fallen to 30°C, it is difficult to detect vital signs such as pulse or respiration. Below 28°C, death is a likely sequel unless warming is begun immediately. The early signs of hypothermia may resemble those of altitude sickness or dehydration It is important in cold conditions to operate a "buddy system" in which travellers look out for such signs in each other.

Treatment of hypothermia

It is not likely that sophisticated methods of re-warming will be available under most travel conditions. The victim should be insulated from further heat loss both above and below the body and sheltered from the cold environment as well as can be achieved. Sharing another person's body heat in a sleeping bag and breathing air in a tent which is heated by the presence of others and by, for example, a cooking stove or heat-emitting lantern are the most practicable methods of rewarming in such situations.

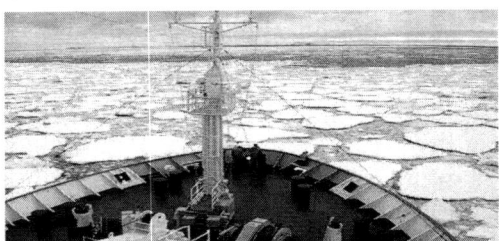

A cruise ship in the arctic

Cold Injury

Frostbite occurs when peripheral circulation is reduced in response to cold conditions and ice crystals form within cells causing tissue damage and, in severe cases, gangrene of the extremities. Affected tissue has a pale appearance and a cold and dead feeling to the touch.

Treatment of frostbite

Affected areas may be rewarmed by immersion in water at or just above body temperature, but if a foot is affected and the victim needs to be evacuated on foot, it is better to allow walking on the frozen tissue before warming, as less damage will be sustained. Re-freezing and thawing must be avoided, as they cause further damage. There is no evidence to support the use of vasodilator drugs. As rewarming occurs, the tissues become red, swollen and very painful and blisters may form. Apparently dead tissue should not be treated radically in the field by debridement or amputation, as recovery may be greater than first appearances suggest. Decisions on radical treatment are best left to a surgeon experienced in the treatment of cold injury.

Frostnip is a less severe form of cold injury in which tissues do not undergo necrosis.

Pre-travel advice
* Ensure that adequate clothing is worn
* Check for the presence of medical conditions such as hypothyroidism which may impair temperature regulation in cold conditions
* Check medication, as many drugs may impair temperature regulation

The older person in hot climates
The reduced capacity of older people to regulate body temperature has already been referred to in connection with cold conditions; it is also relevant to hot conditions19, where it may lead to hyperpyrexia (heat stroke).

A game safari in Botswana

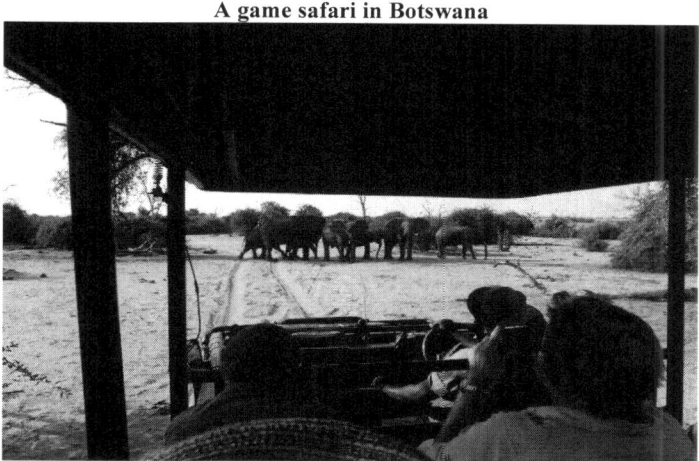

Dehydration
Dehydration, a complication which has already been referred to as more likely to occur in older people12 results from excessive fluid loss due to sweating coupled with inadequate fluid intake. It may be avoided by and adequate fluid intake. Loss of salt also occurs but taking salt tablets not usually needed; a slight increase in dietary salt is usually adequate. Excessive water intake may lead to hyponatraemia.

Heat exhaustion
There is usually a gradual onset. The condition is characterised by a decreased plasma volume and reduced cardiac output which becomes insufficient to meet demands, hence exhaustion. It is caused by loss of fluid and salt. The body temperature is usually normal and always below 41oC. The patient is still able to sweat. Symptoms include fatigue, nausea, weakness, dizziness & sometimes cramps.20

Treatment of heat exhaustion consists of removal from heat where possible, giving oral fluids and cooling, aggressive cooling being necessary if the body temperature is above 40oC (see below).

Heat hyperpyrexia (heatstroke)21
This is a serious medical emergency in which there is a breakdown of temperature regulating mechanisms. The classic "triad" of features is cessation of sweating, a body temperature of 41oC or more and disturbance of central nervous function but the patient should be treated as having heatstroke if any 2 of these features are present. Symptoms may include weakness,

lethargy, fatigue, headache, dizziness, nausea, vomiting, diarrhoea, cramps, anxiety, confusion, unsteadiness or ataxia, impaired judgement, hyperventilation, collapse and convulsions.

Treatment of heatstroke consists of removal from heat where possible, removal of clothing and reducing the body temperature by rapid cooling. Rehydration and maintenance of ABC (airway, breathing and circulation) are important. Evacuation to hospital for intensive care may be required.

Rapid cooling may be carried out by ice water immersion[22] or evaporative cooling using a hammock-like net (or improvising a similar device), spraying with tepid water (not cold water which may shut all directions to facilitate evaporation. Cardiopulmonary bypass has sometimes been used.

Pre-travel advice

* Advise loose-fitting clothing, preferably of cotton rather than man-made fibres and of light rather than dark colour, and remove or replace layers according to the prevailing conditions

* Advise avoiding direct heat from the sun during the hotter portions of the day

* Advise maintaining an adequate fluid intake.

The older person and water sports

Water sports are often undertaken as part of a holiday. They may range from swimming in a heated pool to kayaking and white water rafting in much colder waters. Wherever water is involved in a traveller's activities there is a risk of immersion, drowning or near-drowning and immersion hypothermia.[23] Other risks include ingestion of contaminated water leading to gastrointestinal infection, and leptospirosis acquired by contact with water contaminated with rats' urine.

White water rafting in Peru

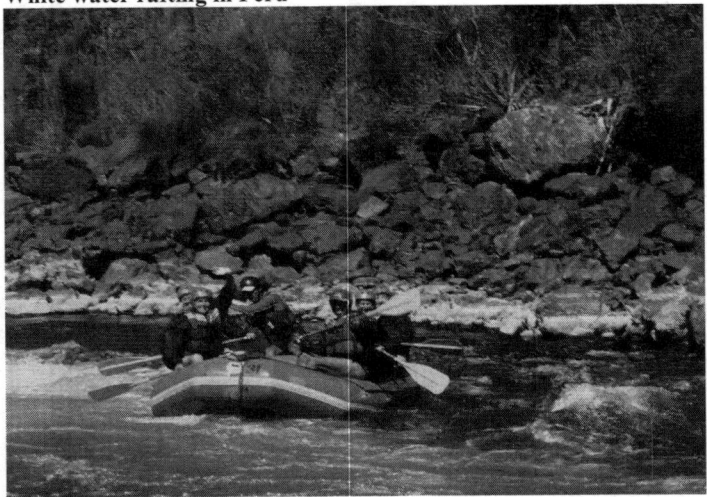

In a study of fishermen in British Columbia [24] it was found that all deaths associated with immersion occurred in water with a temperature lower than 17.5oC, 95% of them in water below 150C. Given the impaired thermoregulatory ability of older people [14,15] it is likely that death would occur in older people subjected to immersion in water at somewhat higher temperatures. However, when the face is submerged, cold receptors in the nasal cavity and face produce an autonomic response that causes bradycardia and peripheral vasoconstriction. This "diving reflex" is not induced when only the limbs are immersed in cold water Blood is diverted from the limbs and internal organs to the heart and the brain, and pulmonary ventilation is reduced. This results in preservation of vital functions and reduces aspiration of water, and is a likely explanation of unusually long survival times seen in some immersed subjects.

Near-drowning incidents and drowning deaths after accidental immersion in open waters have been linked to cold shock response. It consists of inspiratory gasps, hyperventilation, tachycardia, and hypertension in the first 2-3 min of cold-water immersion [25]. This response results in reduced cerebral perfusion and disorientation or loss of consciousness, resulting in drowning. The reduced cardiopulmonary reserve of older people is likely to render them more prone to the effects of cold shock.

The ability to swim is greatly reduced in cold water[26] and becomes progressively impaired as body temperature falls. At a core temperature of 35_0C it is unlikely that an individual would be capable of swimming effectively, and the impaired thermoregulatory ability of older people [14,15] renders them less likely to be able to swim for long periods in cold water unless previously acclimatised to such activity.

A greater proportion of body fat [27] increases the chance of survival, surely one of the few beneficial effects of obesity, and protective clothing also increases the chance of survival. Dry suits have been found to be more beneficial than wet suits in this respect.[28].

Pre-travel advice

* Advise the traveller of the potential hazards of drowning and hypothermia

* Advise the use of reputable providers of water activities with adequate safety standards

* Advice the use of suitable protective clothing such as wet or dry suits

* Ensure that travel insurance covers potentially hazardous activities such as water sports

References

1. http://www.statistics.gov.uk. Accessed 08/06/2011
2. Daily Mail, 24th October 2007
3. http://www.guardian.co.uk/society/2006/mar/08/health.longtermcare. Accessed 08/06/2011
4. Physical activity during the transition period between occupation and retirement. Strobl H. Brehm W. Tittlbach S. Zeitschrift für Gerontologie und Geriatrie. 43(5):297-302, 2010 Oct.
5. Bone mineral density and bone turnover in male masters athletes aged 40-64. Nowak A. Straburzynska-Lupa A. Kusy K. Zielinski J. Felsenberg D. Rittweger J. Karolkiewicz J. Straburzynska-Migaj E. Pilaczynska-Szczesniak L. Aging Male. 13(2):133-41, 2010 Jun.
6. Physical activity, cardiorespiratory fitness and the incidence of type 2 diabetes in a prospective study of men. Sieverdes JC. Sui X. Lee DC. Church TS. McClain A. Hand GA. Blair SN. British Journal of Sports Medicine. 44(4):238-44, 2010 Mar.
7. Master sportsmen. Health status and life expectancies of physically active elderly. Apor P. Radi A. Orvosi Hetilap. 151(3):110-3, 2010 Jan 17.
8. http://www.nepaltrekkinginfo.com/.../trekking/.../everest_trekking.html . Accessed 14/06/2011
9. Acute mountain sickness and ascent rates in trekkers above 2500 m in the Nepali Himalaya. Vardy J. Vardy J.Judge K. Aviat Space Environ Med. 77(7):742-44, 2006 Jul
10. How do older persons tolerate moderate altitude?. Roach RC. Houston CS. Hogigman B *et al*. West J Med. 162: 32-6 1995
11. Ventilatory sensitivity to CO_2 in hyperoxia and hypoxia in older humans. Poulin MJ. Cunningham DA. Paterson DH *et al*. J Appl Physiol. 75:2209-16, 1993
12. Preventing and treating dehydration in the elderly during periods of illness and warm weather. Schols JM. De Groot CP. van der Cammen TJ. Olde Rikkert MG. Journal of Nutrition, Health & Aging. 13(2):150-7, 2009 Feb.
13. www.visit-nepal.com/helicopter-tour-nepal.htm. Accessed 17/06/2011
14. Prevention of hypothermia. McLafferty E. Farley A. Hendry C. Nursing older people. 21(4):34-8, 2009 May

15. Responses to mild cold stress are predicted by different individual characteristics in young and older subjects. DeGroot DW. Havenith G. Kenney WL. J Appl Physiol. 101(6):1607-15, 2006 Dec

16. Injury and illness aboard an Antractic cruise ship. Bledsoe GH. Brill JD. Zak D. Li G. Wild Environ Med. 18(1):36-40, 2007

17. Management of accidental hypothermia]. Hohlrieder M. Kaufmann M. Moritz M. Wenzel V. Anaesthesist. 56(8):805-11, 2007 Aug.

18. Environmental cold-induced injury. Jurkovich GJ. Surgical Clinics of North America. 87(1):247-67, viii, 2007 Feb.

19. An analyisis of factors contributing to a series of deaths caused by exposure to high environmental temperatures. Green H. Gilbert J. James R. Byard RW. Am J Forensic Med & Path. 22(2):196-9, 2001 Jun

20. Exertional heat-related injuries treated in emergency departments in the U.S., 1997-2006. Nelson NG. Collins CL. Comstock RD. McKenzie LB. American Journal of Preventive Medicine. 40(1):54-60, 2011 Jan.

21. Prevention and management of hyperthermia during a heatwave. McLafferty E. Nursing Older People. 22(7):23-7, 2010 Sep

22. Acute whole-body cooling for exercise-induced hyperthermia: a systematic review. McDermott BP. Casa DJ. Ganio MS. Lopez RM. Yeargin SW. Armstrong LE. Maresh CM. Journal of Athletic Training. 44(1):84-93, 2009 Jan-Feb.

23. Management of water incidents: drowning and hypothermia. Dean R. Mulligan J. Nursing Standard. 24(7):35-9, 2009 Oct 21-27

24. How much did cold shock and swimming failure contribute to drowning deaths in the fishing industry in British Columbia 1976-2002?. Brooks CJ. Howard KA. Neifer SK. Occupational Medicine (Oxford). 55(6):459-62, 2005 Sep.

25. Reduced cerebral perfusion on sudden immersion in ice water: a possible cause of drowning. Mantoni T. Belhage B. Pedersen LM. Pott FC. Aviation Space & Environmental Medicine. 78(4):374-6, 2007 Apr

26. Immersion deaths and deterioration in swimming performance in cold water. Tipton M. Eglin C. Gennser M. Golden F. Lancet. 354(9179):626-9, 1999 Aug 21.

27. Two cases of accidental immersion hypothermia with different outcomes under identical conditions. McCallum AL. McLellan BA. Reid SR. Courtade W. Aviation Space & Environmental Medicine. 60(2):162-5, 1989 Feb.

28. Immersion hypothermia: comparative protection of anti-exposure garments in calm versus rough seas. Steinman AM. Hayward JS. Nemiroff MJ. Kubilis PS. Aviation Space & Environmental Medicine. 58(6):550-8, 1987 Jun

Mike Townend

INDEX of CONTENTS

CONTENTS contd